FUNNY YOU
SHOULD ASK

FUNNY YOU SHOULD ASK

A DIARY OF ONE WOMAN'S BREAST CANCER JOURNEY

Tracy L. Matteson

To order additional copies of this book, contact:
Xlibris LLC
1-888-795-4274
www.Xlibris.com
Orders@Xlibris.com
133405

Table of Contents

All beautiful things come from a place of suffering.

To my Mom & Dad, Gee, Samantha, Abbie, Donald, Anneliese and Brian. I love you to the moon and back. I couldn't have done it without you!

ACKNOWLEDGEMENTS

- My three wonderful children, Sam, Abbie and Donald, for "loving me through it", each in your own way, and for your support now, as I "put it all out there" for others,
- Claire Wadsworth, "Gee", my biggest fan, for the constant uplifting encouragement to publish my writing from the second she heard my first journal entry,
- C. Louise Matteson, Mom, not only for her unending support throughout my treatment, but for reliving it a *second* time as my first line editor,
- Brian S. Kelly, my unfaltering paparazzi. The most talented, patient, open and creative photographer and partner I could ever imagine gracing my life,
- My top notch health care providers; without all of you, my experience would not have been the positive experience that it was,
- Rachel Eichenbaum, who instantly came up with the Perfect title for this book!
- Dawn Boyer, not only my friend, but my incredible editor who guided me as I told my story and nurtured my voice through every step,
- *www.caringbridge.org*: Your site gave me the chance to give my journey a voice,
- Garwood, my sweet black lab, who loyally and lovingly lay steadfastly by my side not only throughout my treatment, but during the endless hours of writing and re-writing. Rest in Peace buddy.

PREFACE

IN SEPTEMBER 2011, when I started treatment for breast cancer, I started journaling on Caring Bridge, a website community established for people going through various medical difficulties in their lives. There, they can journal, post updates, feelings, news, and the like, so that friends and family can keep up to speed with their treatment or medical status. As a friend or family member, it's hard to see someone you care about go through difficult medical times. But it's sometimes harder to keep up with how they're doing without constantly calling or feeling as if you're pestering them. Caring Bridge gives patients (or caregivers or proxy family members) the chance to write as much or as little as they want people to know.

After I wrote a few entries for my friends and family, word spread that I was journaling very real (sometimes even humorous!) entries about the realities of breast cancer. Hearing other breast cancer patients say that my entries were helpful to them gave me an accelerated purpose. It felt helpful and satisfying to bond with my other breast-altered peeps. So, I journaled with multiple purposes – as an outlet for me, to keep friends and family "abreast" of my progress, and to give women going through treatment something to relate to, in a positive way. Knowing you're not alone is half the battle.

With this compilation of experiences and explanations, I hope to shed light on the inner worries, battles, and feelings of what a woman with breast cancer may be going through. Mine is only one voice of many. This is my story.

PROLOGUE

Background Story

THERE IS SO much to tell about my journey though cancer treatment. The days leading up to the moment I was diagnosed were when things *really* began, but let me provide you with some background and tell you a little about me. (I'm a talker, so I'll try to make this brief. Wish me luck!) OK, in a nutshell, I am in my early forties, the first born of two daughters, and I possess more of an extroverted Type B personality than an anal-retentive one. After graduating from nursing school, I proudly served five-and-a-half years of active duty as an officer in the United States Navy Nurse Corps and returned to New Hampshire after my tour to raise my family. I am fairly recently divorced, with three downright great kids – two girls and a boy – of whom I share custody with their father. Shortly after my divorce, I bought a house in Northwood, one town over from where I grew up. I am, and love being, not only a mother, but a registered nurse as well. I hold two part-time jobs, one as an executive director, which focuses on more administrative nursing duties (setting up wellness programs for the community), and the other, working in a clinic managing patients on blood thinners. I also enjoy standing in for the school nurse at the local high school when my schedule allows. I am a woman of strong faith. I love to cook and eat well. I go to the doctor and dentist for the recommended checkups to keep on top of my health. I speak fluent sarcasm (the fun kind, not the biting, hurtful kind) and am well versed in non-verbal communication, specializing in eye rolling and the like. I believe that everything happens for a reason and is all part of a greater plan. I try my best to surround myself with positive people and good energy. I am a Sagittarius. I think you get the picture.

Now that you know a few personality traits, let me introduce you to my breasts. For starters, I have always had breasts on the larger side (double Ds, as a matter of fact), and they have always been fibrous. With my medical background as a registered nurse (and a daughter of a registered nurse!), I have always tried to be a "model patient" and have had all things lumpy, bumpy, and irregular immediately checked. Thankfully (to this point), I had always gotten the obligatory, "You're clear. Thanks for checking, thanks for playing, thanks for your co-payment, see you next time, here's your parting gift."

Time and again, I left the doctor's office with ultrasound confirmation that the lump I had noticed was yet another cyst. In fact, I was told once in jest that my breasts had so many cysts that without them, I would probably be an A-cup! The up side of these visits was that with each negative mammogram and ultrasound, I developed a very strong relationship with my OB/Gyn doctor.

All tests were negative until July 2011. Then things got real.

During the summer of 2010, I noticed an area on the outside of my right breast that was painful, hard, and about the size of an acorn. I dutifully made my doctor's appointment and had it checked. As suspected, it was a cyst. This time, due to its size and the fact that it wasn't going away, I had it aspirated by a general surgeon, with a rather large needle and syringe in his office. The contents were sent away to a pathology lab to ensure it was nothing. Thankfully, the results were negative. I was told that if it came back, I should let the general surgeon know. I promised to keep an eye on it.

It didn't *immediately* come back, but about six months after the aspiration, I noticed another lump. Brian, my fairly new boyfriend of a little more than a year and a half, encouraged me to have it checked out, as it continued to get larger and more painful, but I was in no rush. Although I had insurance, a recheck would entail costly co-payments and time out of work for the doctor's visit, and regardless of my OB/Gyn saying, "Better safe than sorry" each time, I felt as if I were wasting people's time. I was the grown female equivalent to the "Little Boy Who Cried Wolf": the "Obsessive Nurse Who Cried Lump." But most importantly, I figured that because it was painful like the last time, it probably wasn't cancer; it was probably the same thing as last year. *Hadn't I heard that if it was painful, that was a good sign, because cancer typically didn't hurt?*

Brian continued to encourage me to have it checked all that spring and into summer, especially when I mentioned that this time, I could actually *see* a golf-ball-sized lump on the lateral (outside) side of my breast. I finally caved and went into my OB/Gyn doctor and had it checked.

My mammography seemed normal, but the ultrasound? Not so much. I had had enough of them to know that this one looked different. Fluid-filled sacs (cysts) are dark on an ultrasound. This one wasn't. The medical sonographer said,

"You had this drained last year?" I viewed the ultrasound screen on the wall and even I thought, *This doesn't look drainable and looks nothing like it did last year.* But what did I know? I wasn't trained to read ultrasounds. Pretty much everything on the screen looked vaguely like a space creature to me. It could very well be some sort of fibrous blob that I wasn't familiar with.

As a precaution, I was scheduled the following week to follow up with the general surgeon, who would review the results with me. Between the follow-up appointment, what I saw on the screen, and the carefully cautious look on the sonographer's face, this visit left me with an uneasy feeling.

Perhaps it's my nature as a Sagittarius, first born, or that I am a nurse, but I am all about preventive medicine, and I like to know whatever there is to know about myself. *What are my lab results? What does this mean, what does that mean?* I want to know how every piece of the puzzle fits together (or what piece is missing), so I can make a "Plan B" in case a "Plan A" doesn't work to fix what's wrong. So, as requested by my surgeon, I picked up my mammogram films and ultrasound report on the way to my follow-up appointment. The front desk receptionist handed me the large manila envelope, and I brought it to my car. But me being me, as soon as I plunked down into the driver's seat, yes, I opened it to read the reports.

I breezed through the benign mammogram report, not fully understanding the level in which the report was dictated, but knowing enough to be able to get a general picture. I then viewed the ultrasound report. Scanning over it, my eyes were immediately drawn to the scary terms that jumped off the page at me. But the line that made my blood run cold was the "impression and recommendations" which read, "**Probable malignancy, recommend a biopsy for further diagnosis**." *Wait. What? That couldn't be right.* I checked the name and date of birth to be sure it was really my report. I was prepared to go to the general surgeon's to discuss a needle biopsy just to ensure this new golf-ball lump was benign like the last time. *Things aren't adding up here. Uggg! Stupid, stupid, stupid! Why did I read this?* There is a reason that patients are advised not to read their medical notes without their doctor there to decipher them. I tried to rationalize through what I read. Maybe they were just saying that it *could* be malignant and that it probably wasn't, so I should have an open biopsy to confirm everything was really fine. *Yeah, right, that sounded good. I'll go with that.* I remained calm, in a numb sort of way, and headed to my appointment.

When I arrived at the general surgeon's office, I handed my packet of information to the front desk before I was escorted to an exam room. And, no, I didn't tell anyone that I read the report. I didn't want to overreact, so I convinced myself that I was probably reading more into it than there was, so I'd just listen to what the doctor had to say. The general surgeon is my age and has a kind bedside manner. I not only trusted, but valued whatever he had to say. He suggested that since the lump they were looking at was rather large, a needle biopsy might not completely represent the contents of the mass well, and it would be more beneficial to undergo a day-surgery procedure, complete with anesthesia, to remove the lump, then send a cross-section of samples to the lab for pathology. *Gulp. This was a far cry from a needle biopsy.* I tried not to be concerned as he presented my options in a very matter-of-fact way; there was no mention of suspected malignancy or any hint of elevated concern. What he didn't know is that I found it very suspicious that he had gone from a relatively minor office procedure to an outpatient hospital procedure. He had read what I had read. Now, **this** was his recommendation. So when he presented it to me in terms of, "If you were my wife, this is what I'd recommend," I knew the open biopsy was the right next step.

He performed the open biopsy on August 5. I had downplayed the fact that I was actually undergoing surgery, but my mom didn't. Although **my** nursing judgment had lapsed a bit, and I forgot that I wouldn't be able to drive home after surgery, my mom's was fully intact. She drove me in and waited there to bring me home. I breezed in and out of day surgery with minimal disruption. After she dropped me off at home and got me settled, my girlfriend Jody arrived. She is also a physicians' assistant, and had volunteered to stay the night with me – just in case I unexpectedly needed something – and we had a slumber party with a glass of wine for her and pain meds for me (win-win!). Brian had left the week before for his annual pilgrimage to Burning Man in Nevada, where he works for two months every summer. Although he was concerned about the surgery, I had encouraged him to leave as planned because, more than likely, it would be nothing, and I was in good hands with Mom and Jody.

It would take about a week to get the results back, and I was scheduled for a follow-up appointment at the end of the day on August 11 to review the findings. Life went back to normal again. I was out mowing my lawn two days after surgery, and other than the inch or so incision on the outside of my right breast, I felt fine.

The evening of August 10, as I waited for my kids to return home from their activities, I wound down my day with yoga. I sat on my living room floor, peaceful, centered, and calm, with a mild curiosity about what tomorrow's afternoon appointment would bring. That evening, all was right with the world.

D-Day (Diagnosis Day)

August 11, 2011

I believe that everything in our life happens for a reason, and that even though God might present it at a time or in a way that we may not understand, it is always divinely perfect. Sometimes, an explanation reveals itself at a later time; other times, we may not ever know why things played out like they did, but it is all part of a bigger plan. Here's an example.

I was scheduled for the follow-up appointment to discuss the findings of my biopsy on August 11. I had decided to work from home that day. In the midst of my morning, around 11 am, I received an unexpected call from the general surgeon's office. The staff there is warm, friendly, and very accommodating. They know me well enough to know that my schedule can be a bit crazy, which had warranted a number of calls back and forth to try to schedule previous appointment times. The woman from the office relayed to me that the doctor wanted me to have a breast MRI as soon as possible, and there was an available slot the very next day at the imaging center in Massachusetts. They wanted to get me right in. She was calling me now to confirm that I could make the appointment. My brain froze. *What? That's tomorrow! Why tomorrow?* My mind couldn't decide if it was whirling or had gone totally blank as I tried to fit all the pieces together. *Was the pathology from the biopsy inconclusive? But wait, even if it was, why would they do a biopsy first and an MRI second to diagnose cancer? Why would they call me now when I would be there in another five hours in person?* It didn't make sense. But instinctively, I said yes to the appointment. I didn't know what it all meant yet, but if the doctor wanted me to have the test, then by all means, schedule the damn test, and I could talk to him about it later and cancel if this was all a misunderstanding, right?

I hung up the phone and put the appointment into my calendar and stood there. Now, what? I was alone with no answers and couldn't call anyone, because I didn't even know what I would say. I didn't know anything besides I had been scheduled rather quickly for an expensive test that was used to pinpoint cancer. Was I scared? Was I numb? I didn't have enough information to feel any emotion, but if I had to spin the "emotion dial," I am pretty sure it would've landed on "anxious." Yep. Anxious won.

Just because I am a nurse does not mean that I know everything there is to know about every medical condition. In fact, I know that there is a LOT I *don't* know, because I am not regularly exposed to it. Although I wanted to remain optimistic that this was all being done in an effort to cross t's and dot i's to ensure it was just nothing, I knew better. The results of the radiology reports that I had read the previous month flashed in my mind. I knew that a biopsy did not need an MRI to confirm if it was cancerous. An MRI is used to see if there is more than the one already identified area. Pathology is pathology. The surgeon excised a big chunk from my breast. It was highly unlikely that the pathology could be inconclusive. It was amazing to me how hard it was to hold on to my medical knowledge when I was feeling like the "patient." If I had been given this information while caring for/treating a patient, I could have put it all in some sort of logical order, but at that moment, all of my logical nursing knowledge danced around in my head somewhere just out of reach. All I could think was, *Is this real? Could this really be happening to me?*

Thankfully, within minutes, the surgeon himself called me. He apologized profusely and said, "I'm sure you are wondering what is going on. The scheduler here didn't realize that I hadn't spoken to you yet, and she was just trying to be accommodating. When I realized what just happened, my heart sank. I know you are a smart woman and you'd figure it out. So, although we NEVER do this by phone, I wanted to call you myself. As you probably suspect, your biopsy revealed that the tissue we removed was cancerous."

He went on to explain a few details and said that he would explain more when we met in the afternoon. He even offered to move other appointments to get me in so that he could answer questions. I said that I wanted to keep my original appointment time. He told me that if between now and then I had any questions that I needed answered, to call the office and have him interrupted. He apologized again before hanging up.

I hung up the phone and sat there. Huh. Cancer. Me. Years of good fortune with my double D twins had suddenly run out. I was about to embark on a journey on the other side of the healthcare world – one as the patient. Holy shit.

Within a half hour, the floodgates opened, and the questions crashed over me. They were unrelenting. *How on earth was this going to go? How bad was the cancer? Had it spread to my other organs? How would they know? When would all of this start? Would I need chemotherapy? Would I need a lumpectomy or a mastectomy and how would my breast look after that? Where would I have this done? How soon would they schedule it? I had a middle-school soccer team to coach in the fall; would they be able to fit me in after the season ended? Would this be the last fall I would be **alive** to coach a soccer team? How would I break this to my kids, parents, grandmother, boyfriend, and friends? Would this be covered by insurance? Would I be too sick to work? If so, would my employer let me go because I couldn't do my job? Would I then lose my insurance as a result? Would I have to sell my house to pay for my medical bills?* The questions went on and on.

After the biopsy the previous week, I'd had the foresight to ask my good friend Shannon to come with me to this follow-up appointment in case the news was not good. If I did have cancer, I wanted to understand the information I was being given before I passed it onto my family; I needed to absorb the initial shock, formulate a plan, and then share it calmly with them as part of damage control. Knowing now that it was truly cancer, I was relieved that Shannon was coming with me. I called her and told her the limited information I knew. Although the news left her somewhat speechless, she offered to do whatever I needed her to. The most helpful thing she could do, other than to be there for me, was to be my second set of ears and take notes during the visit.

If you Google, "What percent of medical information is retained at a doctor's visit?" the number is somewhere in the forty-percent range. Obviously, it depends on the person, the information, and the presentation of the information. Regardless of how this was going to go, I knew I needed someone to take notes of all of the things being said so I could go back and look at them when my head wasn't swimming.

When Shannon picked me up, our first stop was the drug store. I bought a peach-colored composition book and matching folder to document and store everything. Next stop was a local spa, where we had originally planned a massage to relax me before I found out my news. Although I never say no to a massage, I found it difficult to relax fully. I lay on the table wondering what I would be told at this visit, knowing that later that evening, I would have to tell my family I had cancer.

As I mentioned earlier, I was the last visit of the day at the surgeon's office. I knew I'd have his undivided attention. I introduced Shannon and exchanged pleasantries as we were led to an exam room, and he started right in. Tracy, meet Invasive Lobular Carcinoma. So began my "Cancer Patient 101" class.

He drew pictures of lobules (the glands where breast milk is produced), milk ducts (where breast milk travels from the lobules to the nipple), cell activity, the spread of cancer, and why it happens. As the name describes, my cancer was lobular, meaning it originated in the lobules, which are the milk-producing glands, but it had spread into surrounding healthy tissue, making it invasive. If not invasive, a cancer could be considered *in situ*, which means it has neatly remained in the area where it originated. *In situ*, I was told, was easier to treat because of its containment. That figured. He told me about how cancer was staged, explained the process of treatment, and said that they needed a breast MRI to find out the progression of the cancer to determine the course of treatment. If it was in more than one spot, a mastectomy would be required. If it was localized to one area, a lumpectomy would be the recommended course of treatment. His explanations were riddled with many familiar medical terms and occasionally a sprinkle of some that I needed clarification on. It was *not* the time to pretend that I knew what it all meant. It was my time to ask and learn, with him sitting in front of me at my beck and call.

I could feel myself flowing in and out of this surreal environment. I tried hard to push fear aside, to be alert in order to understand everything that was being explained to me, to be present in the moment as though I were in a nursing class learning something that I'd have to explain later to a patient of mine. Only in this case, I would have to explain it to family and friends. I had to decipher what it was that I'd want to share with my kids versus my parents and yet still, my friends.

Shannon's pen was nearly smoking as she jotted things down for the two-hour visit, while I asked questions and absorbed this new information. I had reached full capacity as pictures, notes, and appointments left me with a whirling brain. But for the time being and until we all knew more, my questions had been answered.

I was thankful that things had played out as they did with the way in which I found out about this diagnosis. If I had heard for the first time that I had cancer when we sat down in the surgeon's office, I wouldn't have been prepared. I wouldn't have had the chance to formulate my first round of questions, get a notebook, or really be able to listen. If I hadn't found out that I had cancer until this visit, all of the things that were whirling in my head earlier (after the phone call) would've been taking place at this visit. There is no way that I could have been focused enough to think things through, ask questions, and write things down. I mentioned earlier that everything happens for a reason. I was very glad it played out this way. It was meant to be.

As we drove home from the appointment, my seventeen-year-old, oldest daughter Samantha texted me: "*How was ur appt?*" I didn't see that coming. Although texting is convenient, I knew that this upcoming conversation was one that needed to be in person. I didn't know what to say, so at first, I didn't respond. After a few minutes I got: "*Mom? Ur freaking me out. R u OK?*" I responded with a brief: "*I'll talk to you when I get home.*" Epic fail. Hindsight being 20/20, I knew that was not a reassuring response, and it put her into panic mode. "*Is it cancer?*"

Seriously. I know that texting is the primary form of communication for many these days, but I simply refused to go down in history as "the mother who told her daughter that she had been diagnosed with cancer via text message." It had to be in person. I wanted her to be able to see that I was OK, that I was strong. I wanted to be there to hold her if she cried and reassure her as best I could. I had also wanted to do a dry run, so to speak, with my mom, dad, and sister to see how I would be delivering this news. Absorbing it and saying it out loud were two different things. I felt strong, but I didn't know how I'd respond to everyone's reactions. As a compromise, I told her that I was heading to my mom and dad's, and she could meet me there.

My mom had also made a number of calls to me, checking in to see how things went, and the voicemail she left confirmed that she too was very concerned when I didn't answer during my two-hour meeting with the doctor. After I checked voicemail and noted the "missed calls" on my cell phone, I called her to let her know I was coming over to talk to her, my dad, and my sister, Anneliese. She knew it wasn't good.

Shannon dropped me off at my house; I got into my car and started the ten-minute drive to my parents' house. This visit was going to be brutal. My family was close. And although my mom could make worrying an Extreme sport, she also had equal superpowers to always know just the right thing to say to make me feel better. It's a gift. And yet I wondered, what would she say once she knew one of her children had cancer? I tried to picture myself in her shoes and how I'd feel. Yep, this would be brutal.

When I arrived, I was surprisingly calm. Maybe I was numb. Mom and Dad met me at the door as they always do, with a hug. Tonight's was a little longer and tighter. Anneliese and Samantha arrived shortly after I did. The moments that followed as we went in to sit down in the living room were surreal. How do you act as if you're not about to drop a bomb of information? Everyone's faces were consumed with worry and fear. It was best not to draw it out. As we all sat down in the living room and I had their undivided attention, I said out loud a phrase I had hoped would never leave my mouth: *I have breast cancer.*

To let that phrase resonate in the air felt cruel, so I tried reassuring everyone that I was doing well, considering, and wanted to share everything I had been told. Knowledge is power, right? It felt good to re-iterate what the doctor told me, because I realized that I understood more than I thought I had. One part of me felt confident as the other part of me was having an out of body experience looking down on what was going on. *Was I really having this conversation?*

Samantha sat in front of me, trying to be brave, but cried silently as I knelt on the floor and brought out the pictures that were drawn at the doctors' office and explained what I knew. I reached out to hold her hand and try to make physical contact for reassurance as I continued my explanation to my parents and Anneliese. Samantha told me that after she heard, "I have cancer," everything sounded like the teacher on Charlie Brown (*wah, wah wah waaah, wah wah wah waaah*).

Although it was nice to get our arms around the pathophysiology, even after my explanation, knowing the cellular breakdown of what had developed in my breast certainly didn't address the looming and scary questions that haunted everyone's thoughts. I would have to put my faith in God that everything would be OK. As much as I wanted to know for sure that everything would be fine, only time would tell. Each day, I would deal with what was presented. Mom and Dad were concerned about how I was handling things. I could see that the worry and fear had slightly abated with their efforts to comfort me. Going forward, the verbal exchanges that we shared were questions about next steps, reinforcement that I wasn't alone, and they'd be right there with me with whatever I needed.

My dad reminded me of my inner strength. Only two-and-a-half years ago, I had survived a brutal divorce and made it through that. I could do this too. I was the one who was going to go through all of this, and knowing I had their support and that they had faith that I could deal with anything that would be thrown my way reinforced my strength. We all shed a few tears, but I left that evening feeling calm and secure. The conversation could not have gone any better. Now, to tell my other two children, Abbie and Donald.

Abigail (Abbie), my fifteen-year-old youngest daughter and middle child, and Donald (Don) my twelve-year-old son, the youngest of the bunch, were home when I arrived, as was Sam. After the divorce, the parenting schedule had been split sixty/forty between me and their dad. I was thankful that they were with me and I didn't have to put this off. Before sitting them down, I called and left a message on Brian's voicemail asking him to please call me back so we could talk.

Samantha had already called in reinforcements on her way back from my parents' house, and some of her friends were at the house upon my arrival. I told all three kids that I needed a few minutes to talk to them alone, and we convened in the living room. Although I was trying to keep the tone casual, they all sat frozen looking at me, because it was unusual to hold a "family meeting," and up until then, Samantha was the only child who knew anything about my news. Trying not to scare them, I used my matter-of-fact tone and started in. "I went to the doctor's office this afternoon to review the results of the breast biopsy that I had last week. The not-so-good news is that it is cancer. My doctor told me that I will need a few more tests, and then I will have to have surgery to remove the cancer. Most likely, I will also need chemotherapy and then radiation. I am not sure how soon it will be, but I should know more in the next week or so. I feel fine now and don't really feel any different physically." With them, I didn't pull out pictures or try to explain the etiology, because they didn't care about that. I just presented everything as matter-of-fact as I could, then asked, "Do you have any questions?"

Through eyes welling with tears and a quivering chin, Abigail squeaked, "Are you going to die?"

I calmly and quickly responded, "No." Although no one had told *me* this, and I really didn't know for sure, I hadn't had enough time to even consider death as a real option. And I certainly realized that responding with the more honest answer of, "Jeez, I hope not," would not bring them much, if any, comfort at a moment when they were grasping for any positive glimmers of hope. The girls both asked questions about the treatment. My only answer was, "I don't know much yet, but as soon as I do know, I will tell you." I looked at Donald, who was unsure of how to react. He started out his happy little twelve-year-old self, and after watching the seriousness of the girls' reactions, he figured out that something was wrong, and I noticed him tearing up, too

My phone rang in the middle of the conversation. I looked at the caller ID. It was Brian calling from Nevada. I needed to stay in the moment with the kids, so I answered long enough to say, "I really need to talk to you, but I am talking to the kids now, could you call me back in a half hour?"

Phone calls with Brian were nearly impossible. No surprise, the general reception on the playa (in the middle of the desert) was sketchy at best. His phone battery was unpredictable, being fully charged one second and beeping a disconnection warning the next. His evening schedule varied each night, and then there was the three-hour time difference. Aware of all factors, I knew I had a better chance of talking to him if he called me, because I would be in for the rest of the night, on a phone with a full battery and good reception. He was frustrated and said that he'd try and do his best to call me back, but could make no guarantee. I told him I really needed to talk to him and it was very important. I didn't know if I should just drop the bomb, "Hey I have cancer but can't talk to you right now." Or if keeping him in the dark and letting him hem and haw about the inconvenience of being put off was the lesser of two evils. *Why did it have to be so hard to make the right decision to spare his feelings when all I really wanted was for someone to just comfort ME?* I couldn't hold his frustrations against him. He had called me right away as I asked. But getting my children through this was my first priority.

The kids and I resumed our conversation. Donald took his turn to ask questions. He bounced back to his normal jubilant self and raised his hand as though he were sitting in the front row of a classroom.

"Yes, you, young man, in the front row, what is your question?" I asked.

He said, "I have two questions: (1) Will you still be able to coach my soccer team? and (2) Will you lose your hair?" Both age-appropriate questions from a twelve-year-old.

I told him, "I hope so. It depends on the timing of my treatment, and yes, I will lose my hair."

He nodded and said, "OK, cool." And there ended his line of questioning. I knew that we were all in shock, and I felt the need to be alone for a bit to let feelings shake out. With no further discussion or questions, we adjourned the family meeting.

I encouraged everyone to start getting ready for bed. Life marches on, with or without cancer.

I went to my bedroom and started thinking about what I needed to do next. Like clockwork, a half-hour after his original call, Brian called back. He started by saying that he didn't know how much time he'd have because of the many complicating factors, so I wasted no time delving right into the crux of the conversation. "Thank you for calling me back," I said. "I had my follow-up appointment with the doctor this afternoon, and the biopsy of my breast returned positive for cancer."

There was silence on the other end of the line. Although we could have been disconnected by a dead battery or loss of cell service, I knew he was simply at a loss for words, because I could hear the sound of the wind whipping across the playa into the mouthpiece of the phone. And honestly, I didn't really know what he could say that would make me feel any better. I put myself in his shoes and didn't know what I'd say to me, either.

He and I had been seeing each other for just under two years at this point. Before he had left, we'd had a heartfelt discussion about where the relationship was going. I had wanted to know what was next. Would we continue to live in our own places in separate towns, or would we move in together? I learned that he was happy with the arrangement we had. I wanted more. I decided that our summer apart would be spent doing some soul searching about the future.

Now, this? Perfect. Let's just complicate things more by throwing in a diagnosis of breast cancer, shall we? Would he be able to or even *want to* handle what lay ahead? Would he see this as me "trapping him" into staying with me? I wondered, *What kind of shallow, self-centered asshole would leave a relationship at a time like this?* This certainly wasn't what he bargained for. I couldn't imagine how overwhelmed he must have felt. If he was going to leave, I suppose that now would be the time for it to happen, so I wouldn't learn to depend on him, only to be let down later when he realized he couldn't take it.

But once he found his voice, his words were full of comfort. He said, "I am so sorry. I'm shocked. I don't know what to say. I love you. What do you need from me? How can I help?" I told him I didn't know yet, but that I'd let him know when I knew more.

When we hung up, I was exhausted, both physically and mentally. I needed to do so much. I was starting to make "to do" lists: call my boss, call the insurance company, talk to kids' teachers, get affairs in order. Even though I knew I could take it only one day at a time, I now was placed into a whole different phase of life. One that revolved around cancer treatment as the pivotal point. Everything else going forward would take a back seat.

Tests, Second Opinions, and Formulating a Plan

August 12 through September 6, 2012

My mom drove me to Massachusetts for my breast MRI the next day, August 12. After we arrived at this unfamiliar building, I filled out the registration paperwork and wondered how many more times I would have to do this before it was all over. The relevance of today's test was pivotal. The outcome would determine if I would lose my whole breast, or if I would need only to have a "lumpectomy." As we sat in the waiting room, Mom and I made jokes about the slipper socks and the johnny I had to change into. It made the time go by faster. My name was finally called, and I bid my mother adieu.

I had an IV started, into which they would inject dye, and I was led into the MRI room. The nurse had me disrobe and lie on my stomach on the machine. I scooted myself up to where two oblong holes were located. Through these holes were where my breasts would free fall and hang down and hopefully not hit the floor with an embarrassing "Splat!" (I'm kidding. The machine was a good three feet off the floor.) I was given a set of headphones and a choice of music and was instructed to lie very still while the test commenced. I was told that even the movement of a deep breath would be noticeable on the scan, so I should try to keep taking shallow breaths. Those instructions made me suddenly feel oxygen deprived – it was as if the only thing that would help would be a huge deep breath. With all the control I could muster, I lay still, taking easy, shallow breaths. I tried to concentrate on Carrie Underwood singing through my headphones. When the scan started, I couldn't really hear the music over the noise of the machine. It felt like a long time to lie in one spot, but I wanted to ensure that we wouldn't have to repeat it.

We were told that the doctor there could do a preliminary read. I changed back into my clothes, and Mom and I sat on eggshells awaiting the verdict on the future of my breast. The doctor called us into her little office and showed us the scans and reported that it appeared that the cancer was localized only to the biopsy area. This news meant that I would need only a lumpectomy instead of a mastectomy, followed by radiation therapy. I could keep my breast! Mom and I were overjoyed! She held it together until we were on our way out of the building, when she stopped, held me, and cried with relief. Although I now knew that I could keep my breast, I wasn't as relieved as I thought I'd be, because now a new bunch of questions were plowing full speed into my head about what was next. It all seemed too good to be true. A tumor that was considered "big" at seven and a half centimeters seemed to warrant more than a lumpectomy.

Days later, at my follow-up appointment with the general surgeon, I asked about the process for getting a second opinion. Not that I didn't trust him or the woman who read the report, but I felt that I wanted to do due diligence and be sure I was leaving no stone unturned. "The girls" deserved that, at the very least. He supported my decision and referred me to a major Boston hospital for a second opinion.

I realized early on that I needed to absorb and understand all new information before I passed it on to my family, so instead of asking my mom, I chose to have someone unrelated accompany me to my second opinion. On August 22, I ventured out with my girlfriend Frieda (also a nurse, but, more importantly, that day she was also my second set of ears and note taker) for an all-day consultation in Boston with the "oncology team." This team consisted of a surgical oncologist, a medical oncologist, a radiation oncologist, a genetic counselor, a provider performing a lymphedema study, a phlebotomist, and a partridge in a pear tree. I changed into a gown from the waist up and sat in the room where the surgical oncologist was the first to greet me. She was not only "the" doctor to see, but was also a friend of an orthopedic doctor with whom I work. He said I'd love her. He was right.

She walked in; we exchanged pleasantries and got down to brass tacks. She started with, "**We can treat it; we can cure it**. There is an eight millimeter focus of enhancement less than seven millimeters from the medial margin. Therefore, all treatment options point to a mastectomy as the best option for a cure." *Wait, what did she just say?* Loosely translated, contrary to the preliminary reading of the breast MRI, there *was* in fact a second area of cancer located only seven millimeters away from the larger tumor. I was frozen. I had to stop. The last doctor didn't say that. She said that I would be able to have just a lumpectomy, and that was what I was prepared to discuss at this visit. *How could this be true?* I felt myself getting tearful and felt as if I'd been totally blindsided. I managed to ask, "Why a mastectomy?" She told me, "A right excision/lumpectomy would yield only a ten-to-twenty-percent success rate." To clear the margins, they'd need to remove at least twenty-five percent of my breast, and it is standard practice that twenty-five percent or more requires a mastectomy for the best outcome.

"Lobular cancer is sneaky," she said. "It is known to spread out."

I apologized as I teared up . . . the steel door to my brain had been slammed shut after hearing "mastectomy," and yet it was a no brainer if the success rate of a lumpectomy was only ten to twenty percent. I was in denial as I struggled to accept this plan. Once I pulled it together to try to hear what she was telling me, she explained the details of the mastectomy and the need for lymph node dissection, and then she touched on the options for reconstruction.

However, the one pivotal piece before I could undergo any surgery was to rule out Stage IV cancer. I would need to have a bone scan and an abdominal and pelvic CAT scan to see if the cancer had spread beyond the breast to my bones or abdomen: Stage IV. If it was Stage IV, then the breast would be the least of my worries, and a different course of action would be taken, concentrating on systemic treatment. And there would be no cure at that point. I had been told that the general surgeon had removed seven and a half centimeters of tumor and that the margins were not clear, meaning that the original tumor was even larger and there was more to take. Because this was such a large tumor, she wanted these tests done right away. The doctor reassured me by saying that only around five to six percent of newly diagnosed cancers are found to have spread at the time of the original diagnosis, and that it was "unlikely that it will be anywhere else." Regardless of the statistics, I was now officially petrified. I had an appointment for these scans in another three days. The results could take two to four days. Within the next week, I would know if I had to make plans to put my life on hold for treatment or if I would need to start putting my affairs in order. Fear sucked the breath from my lungs.

I met with the medical oncologist, who discussed the chemotherapy regimen, the radiation oncologist, who explained the process of radiation therapy, and the genetic counselor, who discussed the options for having genetic testing done to determine if I or my girls carried the gene that would put us at high risk for cancer. I had pre-op labs drawn and got the genetic testing done. It felt preventive to know. If the genetic testing turned out positive, I might need to make other decisions, like undergoing a prophylactic hysterectomy and/or oophorectomy (removal of my uterus and ovaries). With the test results, I'd be able to make an informed decision. My mind was spinning and on overload.

I didn't remember much about the drive home. Frieda and I talked about how I was feeling. Other than being overwhelmed, I was exhausted. I had learned enough to scare me all over again. One day at a time.

The night before my scans, I lay in bed and prayed. I pleaded with God. *I know that I am going through this for a reason; that with either outcome, I have a lot in front of me. But, please, I'm only forty-two. Don't let this be the end for me.*

The scans consumed most of the day on August 25. When I arrived at the imaging center, I had to drink two bottles of a chalky drink for the contrast. A gentleman in the waiting room said his daughter was one of the people who had developed the flavors for the drinks. I had to give her kudos. The consistency was really what was so unappealing, and straight vanilla wouldn't have cut it for me. I had the banana and berry flavors. They weren't bad. After drinking the contrast, I had to wait for it to filter into my system.

When I was brought in for the first scan, I had an IV placed. The woman working there told me that they would inject the dye into my vein, and I might feel as if I was having a hot flash in my lungs, then would feel the urge to pee. Sounded like fun. I was very glad she told me, because it was the WEIRDEST sensation I've ever felt. It DID feel like my lungs were on fire, and promptly after that, I thought I was going to pee right there on the table. It was fleeting, though, and over fairly quickly. The bone scan took longer and was scarier. I lay there thinking about what the tech was seeing on her computer screen as the scan of my body slowly appeared. Was she looking at it like, "Oh boy, this one is a goner," or was she thinking, "Yay, another one who is lucking out"? The basic conversations we had gave me no hints of which way she was leaning. She mostly asked me if I was still "OK," because I had to lay still for what felt like a very long time. "OK" had become a relative term.

After a long afternoon, Mom and I drove back home. We headed to Abbie's high school to pick her up and were less than a quarter of a mile from my house when my phone rang. As soon as I answered, the surgical oncologist maintained her positive-foot-forward lead-in and said, "Good news, everything looks great. There is no cancer anywhere else." I held it together, shared with my mom, and tried to concentrate on the remainder of the conversation.

She reiterated that my tumor was large, which meant that there were more cells multiplying and it would continue to grow at a fast rate. Because of that, they wanted me to get right in for surgery. As a matter of fact, they had tentatively scheduled me for September 6, which was fewer than two weeks away! My plan going forward was to meet with a plastic surgeon, and I was given a date to go meet with her. The scheduling got tricky trying to find an opening for both the surgical oncologist and plastic surgeon together.

Then she left me with a question I hadn't anticipated.

"You don't have to decide right now," she said, "but we like to give women the option of having the other breast removed as a preventive measure when they undergo their mastectomies. So, we'll need to know if you want to have a bilateral mastectomy (both breasts removed) as a precaution. It is covered by insurance and often allays the concern of recurrence in the unaffected breast I will need to know if you decide to do so, so that we can book more time in the operating room. It's totally up to you. I just wanted to give you the option."

What? Was she serious? Another decision? I had just barely come to terms with the fact that I was having one breast removed. Now, I was faced with making a decision to remove the other as well? I had heard that this was an option that more and more women were undergoing. The anxiety and stress of worrying about cancer recurring in the remaining breast could be alleviated by undergoing this surgery. Realistically, now was the time to decide to do it. My mind went into overdrive again, thinking of all of the things I needed to consider and get in order before this happened. I was scheduled to meet with the plastic surgeon on Monday. I hoped that maybe she could help me decide from a surgical point of view.

After Mom, Abbie, and I got home, I sat out on the back porch. Mom asked me how I was doing. For the first time, I broke down and cried so hard it hurt. I was overwhelmed with all of these sudden, life-altering decisions coupled with relief. I had been worried that I would have to change my story and tell my kids that although at first we thought my cancer was treatable, the original diagnosis was not accurate and it had spread and maybe I *would* die. The first conversation with them was hard enough. I hadn't allowed myself to go down that fearful path. But feeling that I had narrowly escaped a terminal diagnosis, I was more relieved than I can put into words. I openly sobbed. The tears were cathartic, as though each one released was one hundred pounds of worry freed from my brain.

I called Brian and left a message. Now that I had been given a plan, I had a better idea of what I needed. I knew my family would be there for me, but I wanted someone who could be right by my side at all times. Someone who would be there in the middle of the night if I needed that.

Brian called back. Because I had said that I wasn't sure what I needed or wanted earlier, we revisited the question. I said honestly, "I don't want to do this alone."

He asked, "Should I cut my trip short and start driving home?" I told him yes. He said, "Done," and started making plans to be home in time for my surgery.

I drove down to Boston to meet with the plastic surgeon on Monday. I had a made list of questions, and admittedly, it was strange for me to discuss "new breasts" with her – after all, I had just barely learned that I was going to lose at least one of the pair that I had grown myself and was perfectly happy with. I was feeling conflicting emotions about the prospect of receiving eternally youthful breasts at a time where I had also been given the scariest diagnosis of my life. I wanted to be excited about new, perky breasts (yay!), but that excitement was stifled by the reality that the *reason* I was getting new breasts was because I had cancer (boo!).

I'm a "glass half full" kind of gal, but now, I couldn't tell if my glass was half full, half empty, or if maybe I wasn't even dealing with a glass at all. Maybe it was a plate? Anyway, I started in with a plethora of questions: What were *her* thoughts about undergoing a bilateral mastectomy versus just the right-sided one? What were my options? Would I keep my nipples? And if not, what were my options with that? Would I have sensation? What would the recovery time and restrictions be? What would I wear post-op? What about scars, bathing, risks . . . you name it, I asked it. With each answer, I found my plastic surgeon to be more of an enigma. She was very careful about not overpromising.

She asked me what size I wanted to be, and I said, "The same size as I am now." She said they'd try.

Try. Try? *Why wasn't* that *a realistic request?* When I picture any type of breast augmentation, I think primarily of the surgeries that make breasts perkier and larger. But that wasn't what I was asking to do. I didn't think that asking to stay the same would be an issue. But she would make no guarantees, and I didn't really understand why. I wondered why this piece wasn't as cut and dried as the rest of the cancer plan. I had been held with kid gloves with the rest of the oncology team. I felt as if I were somehow asking for more than I was supposed to.

She did explain that they would take out the diseased breast tissue and put in "expanders," which were temporary "fillers" that would be inflated and deflated as needed, according to the size they would ultimately put in. Expanders would be used to stretch the skin and muscle so that my new breasts would be able to accommodate the implant. They would be filled gradually with saline and would stay in place until after the radiation treatment was done, because radiation can sometimes cause scarring and lead to complications with silicone or saline implants.

I asked to see pictures. She wasn't able to provide me with any examples of situations like mine. This was disturbing, but I was told that she was one of the best. It was time to trust that this wasn't her first rodeo.

She did not offer any guidance as to whether or not she would recommend doing both breasts versus just the right side. Her response was, "It's the patient's preference."

I tried to get statistics: "How many women have both done?"

Again, she gave a vague answer. I would have to make this decision on my own. She said she would see me at my surgery in eight days.

Trying to decide whether to have one or both breasts removed was not an easy one. There were pros and cons to both. The advantages of having only one removed was that it would be less surgery to recover from, and I would maintain feeling in my remaining unaltered left nipple. The down side was, I would have to have mammograms every six months to be sure the cancer didn't spread to the other breast. Lobular carcinoma is more apt to do just that. And honestly, I didn't have a lot of confidence in mammograms, since the last one hadn't identified my very large tumor.

Then there was the issue of asymmetry. Although the surgeons could do a "lift" on the left side to try to equal the right side, after time, gravity would persevere and win over, and I would have asymmetry again. The issue there was that if it bothered me, fixing it would require further surgery, or I would just have to live with it. It seemed that that was cruel and unusual punishment. The advantage of having both breasts removed was that it would alleviate the testing every six months and the anxiety that goes with that, and I would have symmetrical breasts. The down side would be that I would lose sensation in both nipples.

I really didn't know what to do. I asked Brian what he thought. He didn't want to make that call, and I guess I couldn't blame him. But I really wanted a man's opinion. I wanted to be reassured that I could feel sexy after everything was done, but I didn't want vanity to play the leading role in my decision.

So, I put a call into my general surgeon. I respect him not only as a surgeon but as a man who had said to me a month ago, "If you were my wife, I would do the full biopsy." He speaks affectionately of his wife. I wanted to seek counsel from someone who had his pulse on the most current medical treatments and was also a loving husband. I wanted to know what he would recommend if his wife were in my shoes.

When he called me back, I sat on my bed and said, "I know that this is beyond your scope of practice, but I am looking for help with this decision from both a medical standpoint and that of a loving husband. Would you be comfortable with me asking, 'If your wife were in my shoes, what would you advise?'"

He thoughtfully went through the pros and cons of each scenario, but said that ultimately they would do whatever it would take to keep her alive with the best quality of life. Taking both breasts and alleviating the worry of recurrence seemed to make sense. Breasts can be rebuilt, or not. In the end, breast presence or absence doesn't matter to a loving husband/partner. Comfortable that his point of view was coming from a genuine place, I thanked him and hung up, and then made the decision to have both breasts removed.

Now, I needed to put things in God's hands. I needed to find the blessings of each day, because in one week, things were going to change.

I heard from Brian. He had originally toyed with trying to drive back home in his 1970 VW bus, his transportation to and from Burning Man each year. However, with an antique vehicle, it was stressful enough driving when he *didn't* have a deadline, so he made arrangements to leave the bus in Gerlach, Nevada, in a safe spot and fly home. For Brian, this was a labor of love, because he hates to fly. Hates it. But in this case, he wanted to be sure he was back in plenty of time for the surgery. Once I was through the surgery safely and recovering comfortably, he would make plans to fly back to Nevada and drive the bus home for good.

After more than twenty-four hours of layovers and four connecting flights from Nevada, he arrived safely at Manchester-Boston Regional Airport on August 31, less than a week from my surgery. He packed his belongings from his house and moved them in with me, at least for the time being. It was not really how I had pictured it happening, but now was not the time to worry about that.

That Friday, Samantha, now a senior in high school, had a soccer game at Portsmouth Regional High School. I went to the game with Brian and met Jody there. I enjoyed the sunshine and being outside in the stands with the other parents cheering on the girls. They played well.

After the game, I watched their coach bring them in to talk to them. They all listened intently. He then handed each of them a pink rose. "Aw," I thought, "he is so sweet to give them roses." They then walked off to the side of the field to the right of the bleachers where we, the parents, were all waiting for them. I figured that he was moving them out of the sun for a post-game debrief.

But, no. In single file, the girls walked up onto the bleachers, each with a rose in hand. With Samantha leading, one by one, every girl handed me her rose, wished me luck on my upcoming surgery on Tuesday, and hugged me. With all of the parents watching, they kept coming until the whole team had filed through, and I was left standing with an armful of pink roses and tears streaming down my face. Caught up in my own world of questions, anxiety, and acceptance, I hadn't surmised that anyone knew that I was about to go in for surgery. But Samantha had told her coach, and the two of them put together this tender and beautiful moment. Sammy handed me a card that everyone had signed. Parents wished me good luck as they filed out. I was left speechless and moved beyond words. But I clearly felt loved and supported from the members of the team and their families.

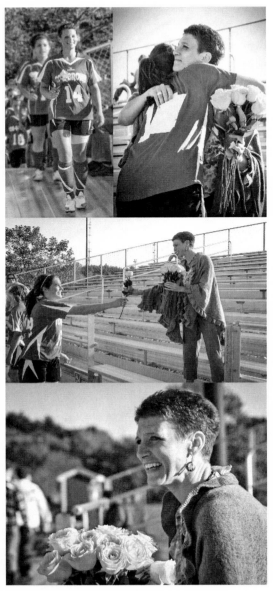

My own version of a rose ceremony

The night before surgery, with a thousand things whirling through my brain about the days ahead, I lay in bed knowing that this was the last night I would have the "function" of my breasts in any intimate way. Trying to push through the worry and sadness, Brian and I engaged in our last intimate night with my body as it was. I made a concerted effort to be in the moment, to memorize the sensation of his touch and the tingling of excitement left from the trail of his kisses. But within thirty seconds, I felt a lone tear escape from the outside corner of my eye. The sensation of that one droplet rolling past my temple and into my hairline opened the floodgates, quietly at first, until I could no longer mask the sobs. As hard as I tried, I couldn't get past the fact that I was only forty-two, and this was the last time I'd have feeling in my breasts. I was just too young for this. I knew that tears were actually quite a buzz kill when it comes to making love. But once they started, I couldn't get them to stop. Brian stopped and held me, and we then cried together. I never asked why he cried, but I knew he hurt because I did. Knowing that was enough for right now. This was the first step toward understanding a different level of intimacy. Ready or not.

I was admitted to a reputable Massachusetts hospital on Tuesday, September 6. I had followed my instructions not to eat or drink anything after midnight, so by the time I got to Boston, I practically had to pry my dry, leathery tongue off the roof of my mouth. I missed my morning coffee.

Traffic was brutal getting in, perhaps more exaggerated by my anxiety. I checked into the nuclear medicine floor, harried and anxious. The staff was clearly used to this level of anxiety, because right away, I was calmed by the forgiving staff at the check-in desk. They ushered me right into where I needed to be without batting an eye, letting me know that everything was fine.

My morning was kicked off with two eye-opening breast injections! Clearly, I would have preferred a nice hot cup of French press coffee to start my day. (Did I mention that I missed my coffee?) The dye would take about two hours to absorb, so it needed to be done first thing, given that my surgery was due to start at around 11 am. After the dye was absorbed into my system, it would "light up" my sentinel nodes so that the surgeons could remove them. The sentinel node is the "first node" in a series of nodes, in this case located in my armpits (axilla). If the sentinel nodes were negative, there would be no further need to take any more. If either of them were positive, the surgeon would remove a larger portion of them to see how far the cancer had gone into my lymph system.

The nurse practitioner brought in two metal vials with the universal yellow nuclear sign on them. That wasn't intimidating at all. OK, I'm lying – that was totally sarcasm. On the contrary, it was extremely unnerving. I looked around, expecting Kiefer Sutherland from *24* to blast in at any moment to tell me that he was "running out of time" to save the world. Instead, it was just me and the nurse practitioner. As she injected the radioactive dye into my breasts one at a time, I was warned, "This might sting a bit." No, the shots of nuclear medicine injected straight into my breasts were not comfortable. But it was time to go with the flow. I had been allowed to take a Xanax a half-hour before I arrived (which marginally helped with the anxiety of the Boston traffic), and I think it might have taken the edge off.

I was escorted to waiting area, where I sat with mom and Brian. I changed into a gown and put all of my belongings in a big white bag with the hospital logo on the side. Brian took a picture of me in my surgical cap and johnny right before I was wheeled off to the pre-op area at 10:45 am, where the anesthesiologists did a paravertebral block. That was no less uncomfortable.

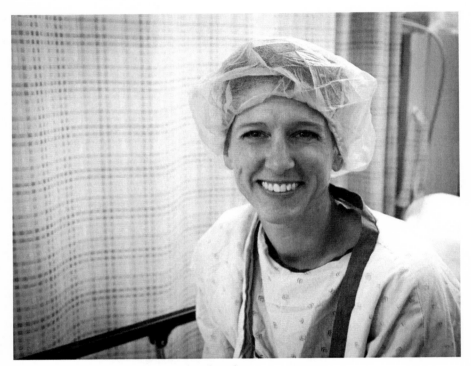

Prepped and ready to go to surgery

I remember the nurses, staff, and doctors all being smiley, happy, and positive when I was wheeled into the OR. After moving to the OR table, I vaguely recall that the last thing I heard was the OR staff telling me that I was in great hands, I would be fine, and that the people there were positive and cared a lot about me and wanted me to know that there was lots of love and healing in the room. As they injected the happy juice into my IV, I drifted off, feeling comforted and calm. I knew I was in the right place.

CHAPTER ONE

My Hospital Stay

Friday, September 9, 2011

ON SEPTEMBER 6, 2011, after a long day for everyone but me (my day seemed pretty short because I was under anesthesia all day!), I hit the recovery room at 5:21 pm. As I tried to acclimate myself while coming out of the anesthetic fog, I was unsure if my paravertebral block had really worked, because although I have never *actually* been hit by a truck, I'm pretty sure that this is what it would feel like. The doctors told me that the block would numb up my chest (not where my nodes were, however) and in turn, I would require much less general anesthesia. The up side was that less anesthesia would lead to less nausea and vomiting. (If this were Facebook, I'd click the "like" button.) It sounded like an offer I couldn't refuse, because really, could there be a down side to less nausea and vomiting? In any event, I was sore, and if this was the extent of the numbness that the block yielded, I didn't want to think about how I'd be feeling without it.

It took me a bit to come out of the anesthesia, and I mostly recall being dry as a biscuit. I was offered sponge lollipops (little sponges on sticks) that were dunked in water to moisten my mouth without absorbing too much water to swallow (and possibly vomit if I had too much). They quickly became my favorite thing *ever.* (Come to Mama, you beautiful little thing!) I was slowly allowed to advance to ice chips, and then I graduated to sips of water.

Upon transport to my room, my newfound friendship with the sponge lollipop was replaced with an even greater love for the not-so-popular emesis bag. I must admit, when I was practicing bedside nursing, there were emesis *basins*. Now, there are *bags* that (unfortunately) I found to be quite convenient, comfortable, and rather user friendly as the motion of transport triggered surges of nausea to wash over me on the way from the PACU to my room. I had a bad case of the bed spins. Once we reached my final destination (thank God the movement had stopped), I wanted to settle in quickly and just be still. But there was my idea of settling in, and the nurses' version of settling in. My version got the kibosh and yielded to vital signs, drain checks, adjusting to a comfortable position, IVs and . . . *holy crap, is it me or is it a thousand degrees in here? Someone turn down the heat, please.* As I was trying to get myself comfortable, my mother and Brian walked in.

At the beginning of all of this, I had asked Brian to document my cancer journey: the good, the bad, and the ugly. He has been involved with photography for a number of years now. Although technically I guess he can't be considered a "professional" because he hasn't been paid for much of his work (yet), he produces exceptional, professional quality work. I felt strongly from the day that I was diagnosed that I wanted people to understand the realities of cancer treatment, whatever it may bring; what better way than to capture it with photographs? So, when he walked in and saw me getting settled, he naturally reached for his camera. It had been no big deal when he took a picture of me in my surgical hat and gown in the pre-op holding area. I imagined that photo being not so much good, bad, or ugly as much as just a ridiculous look for me. But nevertheless, it was real. So, fine, that shot was great documentation. But, now? As a heat wave crashed over me, and a surge of nausea had me grabbing for my emesis bag and dry heaving, I was having second thoughts. Vomiting? Not sexy. And yet the camera was poised and ready. I met Brian's look that asked, "Is this OK?" with a brief shake of my head. Access denied. He instantly lowered the camera. There would be other disturbing moments to capture, right?

Maybe I would regret not allowing that shot to be taken, but at the moment, I wanted my peeps – Mom and Brian – by my side, rubbing my back, handing me a cool cloth, soothing me through my discomfort. Which they did. Thankfully, once I was settled, the nausea abated.

The first night, I was up every few hours . . . vital signs, emptying drains, pain measurements, beeping of the compression boots on my legs (one side pumped up, then released air, then the other pumped up, then released on that side to make my body think it was walking, which would prevent blood clots). The hospital is no place to rest, because healing is a full-time commitment. Shortly after I took pain medicine, and after the nurse took my blood pressure, I was aware of my compression boot going off. I thought, *Why are they taking my blood pressure on my leg?"* Good stuff, those pain meds.

It was tough moving anywhere that first night because I was so sore. Rolling on my side was nearly impossible, and to reposition on my own meant I had to use muscles that I had always taken for granted; it just plain hurt. As I previously stated, my chest felt as if it had been run over by a truck. The surgeons not only cut through muscle but had to do a lot of "scraping" to remove all of the diseased tissue and did so through a pretty small incision. The expanders that were placed in lieu of my breast tissue had to be implanted under my pectoral muscle. I lay there feeling bad for my left breast. I could only imagine it asking, "Why me too? What did I ever do to deserve this? Must I die in vain for the wrongdoing of the cancer that was only in the right breast?" No, that wasn't the drugs talking, I am, in fact, aware that breasts don't speak or have their own feelings. I suppose that it was really that iniquitous seed of doubt speaking, as I was simultaneously hoping that I made the right decision to remove both breasts instead of only the diseased one. There was no going back now.

Around midnight, the night nurse came in to do her assessment of my pain level, drains, Foley catheter, vital signs, and dressing checks. As she reached for the front of my gown to check my dressings, I turned my head to the side and looked away.

"Have you looked yet?" she asked.

"No." I responded.

"Do you want to?" she asked.

I was still trying to acclimate myself to the new room, to the anesthesia wearing off, to the pain, to the occasional wave of nausea, and to the idea that the surgery was behind me. Dealing with those things alone felt enormous.

"No, I'm not ready quite yet," I said. That was OK with her.

But after she left, I noticed my johnny was slipping down further and further, because it had been left untied behind my neck. With my limited range of motion, I wasn't allowed to, nor could I, lift my arms up high enough to tie it. I pulled it up in front of me, but it mocked me and said, "whatever" as it slid right back down again. At that point, I thought, "Well, I'm going to have to look sometime," so I pulled it out and looked down.

It was a train wreck. I wanted to, but couldn't, look away. It looked like two piles of gravel covered by skin. Lumps and bumps and dressings and incisions and wrinkles and, well, flatness. Maybe the anesthesia was making things look this way. I put the johnny back, then opened it up to look again. Nope. It was the same. My not-perfect-but-my-all-mine double Ds were gone and replaced with these gravel mounds.

I have to say, though, that I am very, VERY grateful that I got to keep my nipples. It would have been infinitely harder to look down and not at least see a small something that resembled the former me. (Ladies: If you are ever at a loss for something to wish for as you blow out your birthday candles, I can personally recommend, "I wish to keep my nipples." I don't know for a fact, but I suspect that that is a highly underrated wish.) As much as I dissociated from these small gravel piles, I knew they were all I had, and they would get better. It was time to accept the "new kids on the block." They were only vaguely familiar, but certainly had potential.

At zero-dark-thirty, the gaggle of doctors, interns, and students began their rounds.

I was fortunate enough to be admitted to a teaching hospital. I have never been opposed to being the subject of a learning opportunity. Everyone has to learn somewhere. As a nurse, I used to round with my own gaggle of doctors at the National Naval Medical Center in Bethesda, also a teaching hospital. My empathetic side understood that patients could be daunted and overwhelmed when awakened by a sea of white coats staring, poking, prodding, and asking questions before they had even had a chance to brush their teeth or hair, let alone consume a cup of coffee. But even with that empathy, I still had no idea how surreal it would be to lie in that bed with fuzzy teeth and Phyllis Diller hair, enveloped by that sea of white coats . . . until I was that patient.

The faces were serious but friendly. I smiled and said "Good morning," in hopes that the group could see me as a person. In a teaching hospital, you can quickly become your diagnosis. I was now "A forty-two-year-old, healthy female diagnosed with Invasive Lobular Carcinoma in August, status post-bilateral mastectomy with a right axillary node dissection." Pleased to meet you. It was difficult to remain personal with two-thirds of my bed surrounded by white coasts. I was taken aback when a doctor came over to me, asked a number of questions, and then asked, "Would it be OK to look at your incisions?" *Huh? I suppose that's a rhetorical question.* I lost all nursing perspective and considered the paradox of that question. Could I really refuse? I could have said, "I'd prefer a smaller crowd." Part of me felt like saying, "Have at it, people! It's all part of the job, and it has to be done, right?" The other part was vulnerable and looking for compassion somewhere in that sea of formal white coats. I yearned for a more intimate experience, where someone could acknowledge the enormity of what I just went through. I wanted to expose the reality of how dehumanized and used I felt with a sarcastic comment like, "With all of these people coming to look at my 'boobs,' no one has so much as bought me a drink! I'd even settle for a Starbucks white mocha." Yet all I could utter was, "Sure."

As they carefully took down my gown, I looked down and I saw my own skin . . . only it was a shiny wrinkled mess, with nipples. Even being far less sedated than I was when I looked last night, it was surreal seeing what surgery had left behind in its wake. What I had grown to know over forty-two years was no longer there and in no way resembled what these doctors were seeing. I still couldn't believe it was me.

Somehow, I became less bothered by anyone looking at my chest because, well, it really didn't *look* like my chest, or, for that matter, even a chest at all.

Because I didn't know what to expect, the staff's unchanged expressions and comments like, "Everything looks good," were not particularly comforting.

A nurse practitioner stayed behind to tell me that everything really did look great. I had to redefine "great." It certainly wasn't the great I knew; great was full, double D breasts. This shriveled mess was nowhere near great to me. But she went further to say that she had the advantage of knowing how things would look at the end, after all the final work was done. And where I was looked like the healthy beginning stages of what would lead to a great outcome later. So, in her professional opinion, it *was* great. I hoped she was right.

The two surgeons who operated on me came in separately. When my surgical oncologist, whom I loved, visited, she continued to foster her warm and caring approach. She felt that things went great and reiterated that she was able to remove all of the cancer. We would need to wait to see how many nodes were positive of the nineteen that were removed on the right side.. The sentinel node (I pictured it as the node that donned a military cover and stood watch holding a mini rifle), was positive, which I knew. I would know the results of the rest in about a week to ten days.

After the visit, if it wasn't officially morning, it might as well have been. It was a relief to not have to try to sleep. Because THAT was exhausting! I was hungry after not eating anything substantial for more than twenty-four hours. When my breakfast tray arrived, I was excited, until I discovered that the bedside table where the tray was placed was up so high that when I sat up, I could rest my chin on it. Not a particularly helpful position, especially because I couldn't raise my arms to adjust it. I had to concede, ring the call bell, and ask for help to lower it. I hate asking for help. I got the impression that the staff expected that the patients needed to figure things out on their own. Nurses are busy. And I was happy to do things on my own, but I hadn't been given the green light to even get out of bed, so I really couldn't *do* anything. I did know that my first order of business was to get the Foley catheter removed. I was determined to pee on my own, even if I had to drag myself to the bathroom to do it.

Once I was cleared to get up, although stiff and slow moving, I felt one hundred percent more independent. I could shuffle to the bathroom and wash up a bit. I saw myself in the mirror and thought I looked like a crazy terrorist with all four Jackson Pratt drains pinned to the sides of a rather unflattering utility bra. (The drains look like hand grenades, in case you've never seen one.) Since I couldn't shower, I was thankful that I had gotten my hair cut really short the previous week, so with a little water thrown on it, it looked slightly better than if I had combed it with a chair leg. I had that goin' for me.

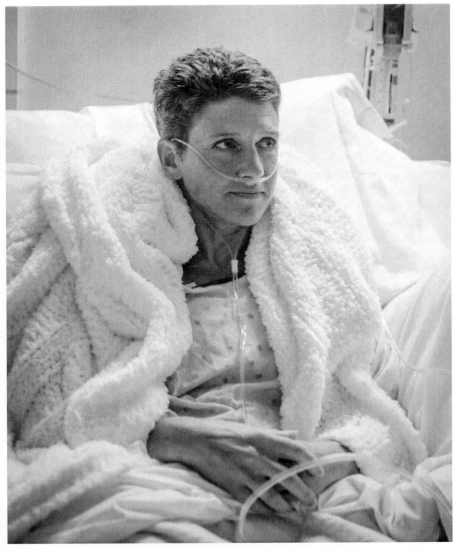

post op day one after surgery

Although they had no real idea of what I'd had to go through to get that far this morning, I was sitting up proudly in a chair feeling as if I'd conquered the world when Brian and my mom arrived. They had been at the hospital all day on Tuesday, only to get to see me for five minutes the previous night. Today, they could spend some quality time. I at least looked somewhat presentable for pictures. And by presentable, I mean awake and not vomiting.

A few friends who happened to be in the area stopped in; I enjoyed their company immensely. Mom and Brian kept me company through the lunch hour, and then, my ex-husband brought all three of my kids to see me in the late afternoon. Don looked nervous. I didn't have time to get the oxygen tubing (nasal cannula) out of my nose before he walked in, with trepidation. I think it was a little weird for him. Each kid carefully hugged me, but his desire to give me a good squeeze let me know how difficult it was for him to see me like this.

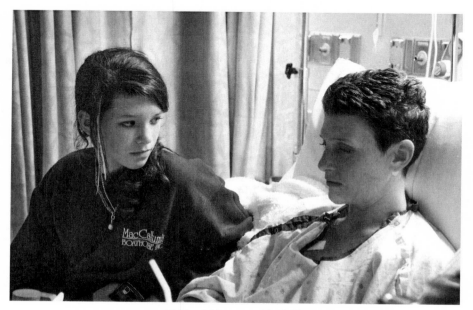

Abbie visiting at my bedside

We all walked down the hallway to a set of couches and visited while the nursing staff got a roommate settled into the other bed in my room. The girls told me I looked thin. I guess I did. Although I hadn't lost any real weight overnight, without breasts perched on my chest demanding their required consumption of space, my frame looked considerably smaller in an unfamiliar, delicate way. The kids filled me in on the details of their days and headed out after a sufficient visit. I tried to remain strong so that they wouldn't worry.

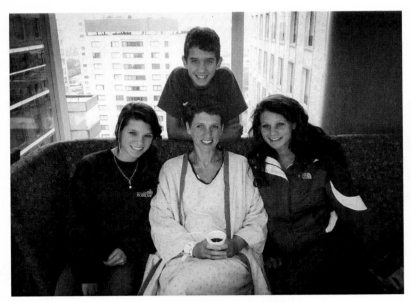

The kids and I post op day one

Everyone stayed for just long enough. I became tired pretty quickly – visiting takes more energy than one thinks. I didn't want to overdo the pain meds, because they tend to make me a bit loopy, so I held off on those until people trickled away. Because mom and Brian had been with me all day, they recognized how tired I had become and headed out with the anticipation of returning in the morning to bring me home.

Although my IV infiltrated that night, and I needed a new one placed for my last dose of antibiotics, the second night was better and more restful. My first post-op day I had checked eating, drinking, peeing, walking, staying afebrile (without fever), and learning how to get along with the pain (not necessarily all at once) off my to-do list. So far, so good. Barring anything going awry, I could be discharged in the morning after my final dose of antibiotics.

After my final visit from the team of doctors on Thursday morning, discharge orders were written, and I was allowed to go home. I didn't see that there was anything that I was doing in the hospital that I couldn't do at home. I was ready.

With much assistance, I got dressed. I had to wear a button-down shirt because I couldn't put my hands above my head to pull a shirt over. Putting on shoes and socks wasn't much easier. As we headed out, I was not allowed to carry anything, which, as a mother who constantly juggles twenty things in my hands on my way out the door, felt weird to me. Placing my seatbelt on the ride home was a bit challenging, but we made it without incident.

Finally getting settled at home felt good, and things felt a bit more normal. The first part of the journey was now complete. The people who stopped in for visits, the flowers, the food, and the cards continued to be uplifting.

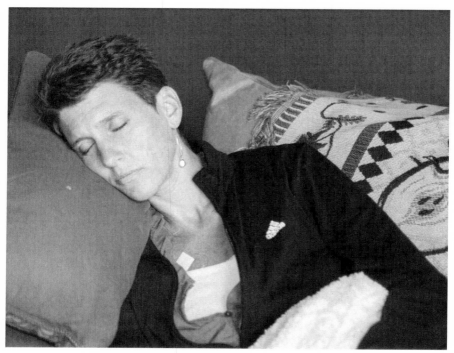

Finally resting in the comfort of my own home

CHAPTER TWO

The Challenges of Recovery

Tuesday, September 13, 2011

S O, YOU ASK, how hard could all of this recovery stuff really be? Well, let me tell you, it's waaaaaay harder than I ever expected! And the challenges are not all physical, either. So here's my first week home in a nutshell.

As planned, after I was home and settled for a few days and comfortable, Brian flew back out to Nevada to pick up his VW bus and start the drive home. It would be a six-day drive with a top speed of fifty, even with the tail winds pushing him, barring any unforeseen catastrophes. He checked in at least daily. Although it sounded like an adventurous experience, after hearing about how he was living off of truck-stop food, sleeping in his van, and using only public restrooms for five days, I was thinking that recovering from surgery sounded like a heck of a lot more fun. At least I had good pain meds and people bringing me dinners! In his absence, Mom offered to stay with me to help me out as I slowly gained back my independence.

I will start off by saying that the key ingredient to keeping my sanity was largely due to the support I was surrounded by. I don't know that I could have done it without not only my mom, but my friends and family close by, literally at my beck and call.

A week out of surgery, "the fear of the unknown mastectomy" chapter was behind me. Questions like, "What will I look like?" "How will I feel?" "What will my limitations be?" were being answered. But as an active person who generally has about thirty things going on at once, ninety percent of which are voluntary, this recovery stuff hit me upside the head and smacked me into reality.

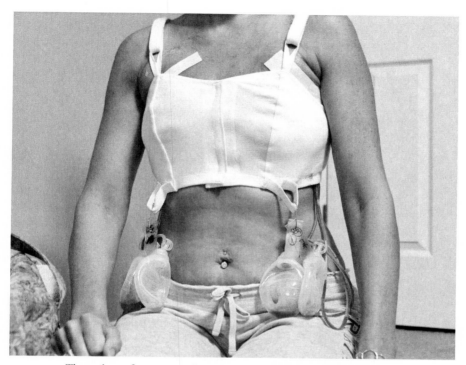

Three days after surgery. Drains, dressings and surgical post op bra

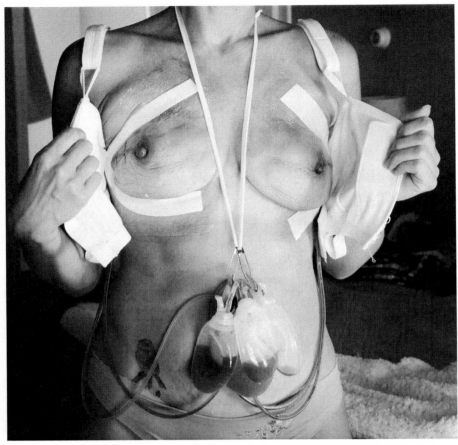

The reality of what I looked like after surgery

I received post-op calls from the hospital nurses. They provided me a chance to ask questions or report any abnormal findings. Thankfully, my responses were pretty benign. And, don't get me wrong, there was a lot going on, but to mention it to them might have sounded like whining.

I'll whine here.

Living with the four drains was no fun at all. I had been counting down the days until my first follow-up appointment, because I could have them removed if they had 30 cc or less of fluid in a 24-hour period. They needed to be emptied twice a day, morning and evening, when I recorded the output on a flow sheet. After I emptied the first drain, I realized that I had left the flow sheet in the kitchen. I quickly turned around from the bathroom counter to head back to the kitchen to get the paper and was stopped dead in my tracks by a sharp pain in my side. The tubing (going from the drain into my side) had wrapped around the doorknob and pulled the door closed behind me as the stitches that held it in my body stretched to capacity. I briefly saw stars. Those things could not come out soon enough!

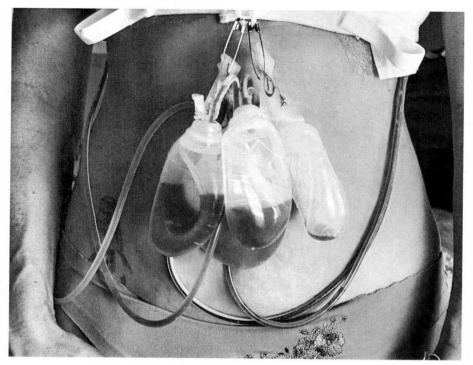

All four drains

Over the past few days, I had two drains with minimal drainage and was quite pleased. I assumed they'd be pulled when I went in on Monday, and that would cut the number of drains by half. But on Sunday, one of those two drains decided to kick it into high gear and set some new output records. I don't know that I did anything to make this happen; my body just decided that it needed to do it. I knew that now there was only the chance of one being pulled. I wanted them all gone. Very discouraging.

Monday morning, I got dressed up in a work button-down blouse and capris to go to Boston for my post-op check. Dressing up has always made me feel better, no matter what the occasion. But I now found that nothing fit. The drains and lengths of tubing hung down off of the bra they gave me and landed right around my waistline. Hiding them inside my blouse made me look pear shaped. Accentuating that further was the fact that where there used to be breasts, there was virtually not much of anything at all. How to feel feminine and put together when nothing fit or felt flattering was a transition I had not expected to experience. So, I wore my faux-pink, alligator skin, pointy-toed heels to detract from the upper half of my body. That actually seemed somewhat successful.

Once we arrived at the post-op appointment, I had only the one drain pulled, as I'd feared. (Damn it! I was hoping for at least two!) And had I not come with a list of fifteen questions, the appointment would have been less than five minutes! When the drive to Boston is an hour and a half, parking and making your way to the appointment is another twenty minutes, and the wait is yet another fifteen minutes, it feels anti-climactic to go in, have a drain pulled, and get a "See you in a week" before the doctor leaves. *Seriously? Hang on a second, doc . . . can't we talk about how fabulous I've been doing or at the very least how I'm rocking these shoes? Give me some love, some affirmation, some kudos. Something!* Didn't she understand how hard it was for me to be still and let others do things for me for a whole WEEK? Had she forgotten how many restrictions this surgery had put on me over the last few weeks – no lifting, no driving, no sex, no raising my hands over my head, no housework – not to mention that sleeping with these wretched drains was near to impossible, I was overtired, couldn't poop because of the pain meds, and was trying my best to keep a sense of humor through all of this? *Could you please throw me a bone here?* Alas, no. If she did know any of these things, they were certainly not her primary concern.

I did have a chance to ask questions, but even the answers to those were discouraging. It sounded as if they had to make more incisions than I had originally thought, and I didn't understand why. I might not be able to return to the same size I was pre-surgery, and I couldn't comprehend why that was, either. I'd be OK if I ended up a little smaller, because I supposed the perkiness would make up for size, but I hadn't anticipated that they may only be able to get me within TWO cup sizes of my normal size. This was information I would need to digest. And no matter how many sneaky ways I asked about getting back to my normal routine, the doctor still told me I needed to take it easy and wait "four to six weeks." She wouldn't budge. I even tried asking her in pig Latin, thinking I'd get a different answer . . . but no. Still *our-fay to ix-say eeks-way of ecovery-ray.* $#!+! I get it. My body needed it. I am no Lindsay Wagner. I am only human. One would think that going into the original surgery in good shape with a body I had taken good care of would give me a little bit of a head start and perhaps shave off a little recovery time. Sigh. Not so much.

So, I found that the days of my appointments were my "down" days. I had to hear what had to be said, then absorb it, feel how I felt about it, and just sit with it for a bit. By the next day, I'd have a better level of acceptance and be more able to put a plan together, look at the bright side, and figure out how to move forward. I worried about people contacting me on those "down" days, because I even *sounded* down. I didn't want people to think I was perpetually down and discouraged. So, I tried to keep interactions with the outside world to a minimum on those days.

I hoped the final pathology would be back soon. They told me it would take seven to nine days. They had already told me that I had cancer in my lymph nodes, which wasn't a surprise. It essentially put me at a Stage III, but I hadn't yet been told that officially. Once the pathology was back, I would reconvene with the entire oncology team in Boston, and they would outline a treatment course for me. They prepared me for the possibility of needing both chemo and radiation, although I didn't yet know for sure. Both sounded as if they'd be safe to undergo, and they'd decrease the chance of recurrence later on. If I could arrange for that meeting on Monday when I went back for my next post-op check, I could kill many birds with one stone. I hoped to be able to receive the chemo and radiation therapy in Dover, NH, a town close to where I live and work.

My pain was still present, and I had a plethora of good pain meds to help me through that. However, they led to problems in other areas, which led to worse experiences than the surgery pain. Namely, constipation. (And all of the fun that goes with THAT bundle of joy!) The bummer (no pun intended!) is that I *knew* this complication was a possibility. I started ON MY OWN back when I was hospitalized, asking nursing staff for stool softeners to counteract the pain meds so I wouldn't run into this *very problem*. Yet, alas, I was not proactive enough. As if everything else I was dealing with wasn't enough, now (OK, brace yourselves, I'm just going to say this) *pooping* had gone to the top of my list of problems. (Glamorous, right?) Seriously, I'm too young to be discussing my bowels. But, I can see now why life can revolve around pooping. It became a topic of conversation because I didn't want to eat until I went, and I developed a love-hate relationship with the bathroom; I was hopeful and scared at the same time that each visit would "be the one." It goes without saying that it all put me in a rather foul mood. What an ordeal.

The other really fun challenge was that I still couldn't move my arms more than ninety degrees up in the air. So, I couldn't get to my coffee cups, dishes, or anything else that was not already on the counter. I had the step stool close by, but I wasn't supposed to lift more than ten pounds, either. It seemed that everything suddenly crossed that threshold. Yet, I learned to anticipate the problems, accommodate what I could, and let the rest go. I left a complete set of dishes on the counter so I wouldn't have to reach up to get them. When the hook from the shower curtain came off the rod, and I couldn't simply reach up and fix it although it taunted me after I eyeballed it, swore at it, and willed it to go back onto the rod on its own (which it didn't), I had to *ask* someone to do it . . . . Gah! I suck at being dependent.

I was TOTALLY blessed with meals for dinner every night and beautiful bouquets of flowers to brighten up my days. Friends brought magazines, lunches, books (dirty joke books!), and movies. They offered rides and button-down shirts. People I hadn't heard from in ages resurfaced to show their support.

There are blessings with cancer. People's good sides come out, and they step up and do things without batting an eye. Whether it was a meal, a laugh, or even just an encouraging text message, I enjoyed this part of recovery.

Upon his return, Brian continued to document my journey with photographs. Barring the mid-word photos (yes, even recovering from surgery, I talked a lot, which made it difficult for him to get a good shot of me), what he captured might be sad, medical, emotional, or happy. Although they wouldn't all be flattering, they would be real.

Each day was different. Some weren't so great; some would be better. I tried to notice when a day was beautiful. I willed myself not to push too hard, and I tried to nap when needed so I could save my energy for my family and friends. I hoped that each day would bring more strength and good energy.

CHAPTER THREE

Next Steps

Thursday, September 15, 2011

I HEARD FROM my surgical oncologist. She is well versed and a straight-A student in the School of Optimism. With an upbeat voice, she always started off her conversations on a positive note. She reported to me that my pathology results came back, and although the right breast had cancer throughout, it was not anywhere near the nipple, which reinforced that performing a "nipple-sparing mastectomy" was the best choice for a cure. She confirmed that the "margins were clear," which was great news. Although cancer on the left breast had already been ruled out by mammogram and ultrasound, all of the breast tissue they removed was sent to pathology, double-checked, and officially declared to be cancer free, so no surprises there. (Phew!)

The right sentinel lymph node, however, was positive for cancer cells, as we had known from the frozen section taken during surgery. I'd been prepared for that finding because my tumor was so large. So they took a total of nineteen nodes. Besides the sentinel node, there was one node with micrometastasis and another node with macrometastasis. Micro means the node had a < 2 mm area of cancer, and macro means > 2 mm area of cancer in the node. So that was three out of nineteen . . . it could've been so much worse. This was great news.

I had an appointment with my plastic surgeon on Monday at 10 am, where she would remove my dressings for the first time and (I hoped) remove the remaining three drains. In addition, since we had a positive pathology report, I also had an appointment at 8 am with the medical oncologist. At this appointment, we'd discuss when the chemotherapy regimen would start, what drugs I would receive, how frequently I would receive them, and where I would – and could – be treated. As wonderful as these Boston doctors were, I wanted to be closer to home if possible. Heading to treatment would be more palatable if I could sip on coffee and have a straightforward commute of a half-hour to the local cancer center, as opposed to the unpredictable one-and-a-half to two-hour commute to Boston.

We would also discuss more about the hormone regimen I'd receive. I was told that hormone therapy reduces the risk of recurrence by forty to fifty percent! There is really no other area of medicine that can improve an outcome like this. The only down side to hormone therapy was that it would make me feel as if I were going through menopause. (Yeah! Good times!) But it would have such a positive effect and outcome that it would be crazy not to endure it. Bring on the hot flashes and the crabbiness!

Meanwhile, back at the ranch . . .

Although I was generally NOT a morning person, mornings became my best time, where I had the most energy. By noon, I was ready to nap. Afternoons were pretty slow and steady. One day, I got up and went for a short walk around the block with a neighbor, and although I had big plans for going to a soccer game that afternoon, the weather turned cooler, and the last thing I needed was to be cold and wet and then come down with something miserable in the midst of all of this! So, regrettably, I decided to take care of me and sit this one out.

The kids spent their first few nights back home after being away for more than a week with their dad. They had visited, but had not spent the night. They were great about getting supper ready and cleaning up afterward. So many generous friends and neighbors brought food that we were grateful to be able to just "heat and eat!"

I will share the following about the physical part of my recovery:

Warning Number 1

Medical Information Ahead (Not for the Faint of Heart)

I became aware that my drains were not draining well, and I was becoming physically uncomfortable. I noticed fluid accumulating in a rather large pocket under my skin, which was also mentally uncomfortable. This is where being a nurse came back to bite me. I started thinking about every possible thing that could be happening and worried about how it would impact my overall recovery.

Is there a clot lodged against the end of the drain, causing this serous accumulation? What if it festers and then becomes infected? Will that damage my skin? Will I need IV antibiotics or can it be treated with oral antibiotics? Crap. Now, I'll surely end up with a raging yeast infection from the antibiotics. Mental Note: Ask doctor for prescription-strength Fluconazol to cure the yeast infection. Is this worthy of a call to the doctor, where she will say, "We're glad you called, nice catch"? Or will she roll her eyes and say, "Krikey, lady, just relax, it will naturally reabsorb and you'll be fine"? Gah! Being a patient was HARD! I was all set to call the doctor, but after my shower, I must have dislodged a clot or something, and the fluid drained like crazy. So, that seemed to resolve itself. Ahhhh! This was a win-win for me – no infection, no antibiotics, and no yeast infection! Even though I made it all up in my head, I still felt as if I dodged a bullet there.

Warning Number 2

Disturbing Reality (Not for Those Who Are Queasy)

Because I wasn't allowed to lift my arms to shave my armpits after surgery, I'd soon be able to braid my underarm hair. Seriously. Everything about that was just wrong. And definitely not sexy.

And *speaking* of not sexy, let me shed a little light on my clothing dilemma. I equate this fashion frustration to the awkward "in-between" stage after you've had a baby, but before you've lost the baby weight. None of your pre-maternity, "normal" clothes fit, but your maternity clothes just hang off you like a burlap bag with no form or style; at best, they look frumpy and disheveled. As I experienced when I went for my first follow-up appointment in Boston, for me, it was hard to feel pulled together when nothing fit right.

As I have mentioned a thousand times, I wasn't allowed to lift my hands over my head; therefore, for the time being, my options were button-down shirts. Period. My selection consisted mainly of those I wore to work, and they were on the dressier side. I didn't have any outside of this category. In light of this fashion emergency, my mom, sister, and my friend Shannon brought over a few of their tops for me to borrow. Not only were they easy to get in and out of, but I had no predisposed ideas of how I should to look in them the way I did with my own clothes. It was hard to don my favorite shirt just to see it swimming on me where my chest used to stand out. (*Et tu*, purple button-down blouse?) I'd come to expect to look a certain way when I wore my clothes, and when I didn't, well, it felt like yet another thing I had to give in to. I was reminded of the reality – my breasts were gone.

It's not as if I could *ignore* the fact that they were gone. I wasn't in denial. I knew that being breast-less was part of the deal, and for that matter, I knew it was temporary. But at the end of the day, the reality was, *knowing* they were gone didn't make it suck any less. I missed them and all their glory. But, I think most of all, I missed feeling complete. I shared this frustration with Shannon when she dropped off her shirts one afternoon. (God love her. It's a gift to be able to know what to say to *that*, right on the spot.) She said that although I had always been big-busted, maybe now was the time to embrace all other phases of "breasthood," if you will, and try them on for size. Perhaps I just might find that long-forgotten, A-sized breast now sitting upon my chest to be "sporty." Huh. Sporty. Sporty was good. Sporty was respectable. In many cases, I was pretty sure that sporty was even sexy. I thought that she was onto something there. Maybe I *could* rock each of these cup sizes as I made my way back to my size. *Occupare Pectus Mole*: Seize the Breast Size. (It's no *Carpe Diem*, but it just might catch on.) I would start by rocking my sporty size A.

So the borrowed tops alleviated any preconceived notions of how I was *supposed* to look, and my new outlook on embracing each breast size, believe it or not, really helped me. The shirts were new (to me), and my chest was new. I could do this.

CHAPTER FOUR

Onward, Outward, and Upward Progress!

Wednesday, September 21, 2011

S O, YES, THIS title is an attempt to be witty. I received a ton of information about my next steps (onward), had my first "fill" in my expanders (outward), and learned a few lessons (upward).

Monday, I had a big day planned, and it started early in Boston at 8 am with Brian, who arrived home safely the past week, and my mom. But no matter how I tried to plan things, we'd leave just ten minutes too late to get to the hospital on time. Boston traffic is unpredictable, and this day proved to be no exception. We hummed along quickly on Route 93, but once we hit the exit for Storrow Drive, we were essentially at a standstill. I watched the minute hand tick away as we crept along the last two miles to the hospital. I decided to try to call the Oncology Floor to let the doctor know we were going to be about five minutes late. I dialed a main number that connected me to an operator who, evidently, hadn't finished her morning coffee and was irritated that I would dare to call before 8 am. She told me that there was no doctor by that name at this hospital. *What? Yes there is; she's not only well known there, but I recently saw her!* I spelled the oncologist's name, gave her the department, and tried to tell her that I was going to the cancer center. Her responses to my apparently unhelpful information became increasingly irritated. I finally asked if there was an Oncology Department number she could try, and she abruptly transferred me. I breathed a sigh of relief when I heard a recording that said that if I wanted to leave a message, please stay on the line. Finally, some progress! After a minute of music, I was transferred, yes, you guessed it, back to the surly operator! She all but yelled at me. "I JUST SPOKE to you and TOLD you that there was no doctor by that name." I personally couldn't imagine speaking to anyone like that. I guess I should have gotten her name, but instead, I contemplated what to say from all of the responses swarming around in my head. *Look lady, I'm just a newly diagnosed cancer patient, trying to be mindful of the time schedule my doctor is trying to uphold. I wanted to let her know I am going to be a little late. I am very anxious about what is going to happen today, and I don't need or appreciate your* sass *this early in the morning. It's a good thing I already know and love this hospital, because you are the first person people speak to, and therefore, you leave the first impression for this hospital. If I had to rate you, I'd* maybe *give you a one on a one-to-ten scale and then send you straight to anger management class. If someone peed in your Cheerios this morning, you don't need to take it out on me. And one more thing . . . your mother was a hamster and your father smells like elderberries!*

Instead, I swallowed hard, said, "Thanks for your time and have a nice day," and hung up. After that, the cork exploded, and I shared my entire bottled-up inner monologue with my captive, commuting cohorts, Mom and Brian. Even though the operator couldn't hear it, boy did I let her have it! It felt good to get it off my chest. Perhaps some of my ranting was driven by the fact that at every turn, I prepare for the worst and hope for the best. Yet there I was, stuck in a car, feeling out of control, not only because I was late but because I was heading into an appointment to discuss the scary stuff – the chemotherapy – then go through a new and unfamiliar procedure. But mostly, I think the operator was crabby.

I met with the medical oncologist a few minutes past 8 am. Now that we knew my stage of cancer from the results of the lymph node dissection, we could put together a real plan. I was officially Stage III because of the size of the tumor and the fact that there were lymph nodes involved. Mom, Brian, and I all talked with her, or actually, mostly listened to her, for more than an hour.

This is what I learned.

The medical oncologist told me that the recommended treatment would be chemotherapy every two weeks. The first four doses would consist of two drugs, and the remaining four doses would be a single drug, all administered by IV. The up side was that it sounded as though the days of terrible nausea and vomiting from chemo are days from the past, because now there would be a "cocktail" of four drugs that would take care of that. The down side was that they cause constipation, which can be worse than the nausea and vomiting.

Now, perhaps you are young enough, or simply lucky enough, to not have experienced what it's like to have "bowel issues." Good for you . . . really. We roll our eyes when we overhear older family members or acquaintances talk about their habits, what they take for it, and how the results all come out. Gross. TMI. But I just have to say, when you are a "regular" girl and this gets out of whack, it's as if the stars and planets are out of alignment. Nothing feels right until "Uranus" is back in orbit. I will not give details, but let's just sum it up by saying that I have learned the mere MENTION of narcotics causes my intestines to seize up, and all peristalsis comes to an abrupt stop. And it is an ordeal and a half to get things right. I say this because, well, I was looking at two pretty crappy (pardon the expression) options: nausea and vomiting, or constipation. I would need to be diligent to keep both under control during the first four treatments.

The doctor also told me that I would receive a shot twenty-four to forty-eight hours after the chemotherapy infusion. It would keep my white blood cell counts high enough to not dip down to scary levels. If the levels dropped, I could not receive my subsequent treatment. I was told that the chemo I would be receiving rarely drops platelets or white blood counts down to scary levels, but that may be because this injection is used. The side effect of this injection is that the after effects are painful in the bones and joints. Pain is subjective. Some say, "It's an ache"; some say, "Nope, it's PAIN!" I would have to experience it myself to figure it out. But I felt better being prepared.

She went on to explain that in fourteen to seventeen days, like clockwork, I would lose my hair. All hair. Seriously, as intimidating as that was, because I couldn't shave after surgery, my underarm hair was now officially out of control. This fact compounded an additional conundrum; I was not supposed to use deodorant, either. However, I was told that I could get an electric razor and use that, but at this point, was it even worth it? And really, how disturbing is it to picture an electric beard trimmer plowing through a forest of armpit hair?

She told me that one thing the books don't really mention is that the hair loss can also hurt.

Please don't get me wrong. As much pain as she described that goes with this treatment, this doctor was tender and caring, and was only filling me in, as gently as she could, to be sure that I was fully prepared. Because of her gentle presentation of all of this information, it wasn't scary to hear. The only thing I feared was that I would forget something important that she told me about. And for that, I had my mom taking notes.

In every dark situation, there's always good news that shines a little light. A nugget, something that makes you think, "Well there, at least there's that." In my case, it was hearing that some women cease menstruation during chemo and then after for about nine months! *A respite from menstruation? Is it my birthday? This is my silver lining!* That news didn't break my heart. What a nice little bonus! Although I was told that I may have hot flashes and perhaps a mood swing or two, I was OK with it. I was forty-two years old, and my child-bearing years were over. That ship sailed after my sweetie son was born, and I am happy and blessed with three beautiful children.

After the first eight weeks of treatment, the second eight weeks change to a single drug. This one does not cause nausea and/or vomiting, so I wouldn't have to worry about taking the drugs to prevent it . . . only about the drug itself. Two days or so after the infusion, this drug would cause my body to . . . . you guessed it . . . be in pain. More bone pain, joint pain, all-over general pain. Only for a few days though. In both treatments, there would be a few bad/down days and then things would return to fairly normal. I was good with that.

I decided to coordinate with my local hospital to have the treatments closer to home. If I could have transported my doctor to New Hampshire, I would. She was lovely and very positive. (And laughed at my jokes and liked my shoes . . . which can make or break a doctor-patient relationship!) But the commute to Boston and fighting traffic ranked up there with constipation. So, as much as I loved her, I would stay local so I wouldn't have to add hypertension to my list of medical issues that would result from the anxiety of fighting Boston traffic.

The chemotherapy could start anywhere from four to six weeks after surgery. Four weeks would put me only two weeks away from a start date, if I could get right in. I didn't know how it would work.

After that appointment, I went to the plastic surgery floor for my first "fill." This is where an ARNP would begin weekly injections of normal saline into my "expanders" (aka gravel piles) until I was a size or two above where I would be after reconstruction; roughly when I could fit into my old bras. The expanders would stay in until after all treatments (chemo and radiation therapy) were done. Their purpose was to create a place to put the permanent implants by stretching the skin and muscle before I went in for my final reconstructive surgery.

They had me change into a gown, and a medical assistant checked me in and took down my dressings and redressed them and pulled one more drain. A nurse practitioner came in and walked me through what she would do. She had a little one-inch instrument with a magnet that she ran over my breast. Evidently, there was a metal piece in the expander that pulled the magnet, which allowed the practitioner to find the spot to inject the saline. (It reminded me of how, as a kid, I'd try to find water by holding a Y-shaped stick out in front of me, and it would bend down in the presence of water.)

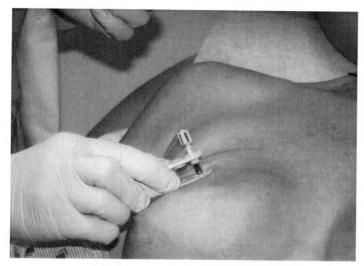

The magnet used to locate the port

When the magnet attached to the area, she pressed down on it, and it left a little "x," which marked the spot. After a quick swipe with a Betadine swab followed by an alcohol pad, she put the needle into that spot.

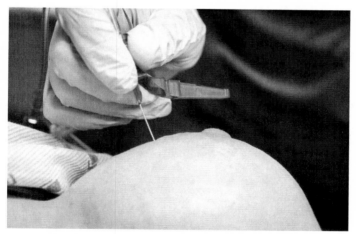

The needle goes in

I had no feeling in most of the areas of my breasts because so many nerves were cut during the surgery; so, thankfully, I didn't feel anything as the needle went in. The nurse practitioner then pushed in 60 cc of saline (equivalent to two ounces or a quarter of a cup of fluid). I watched my virtually flat chest take shape before my eyes as she slowly injected the fluid.

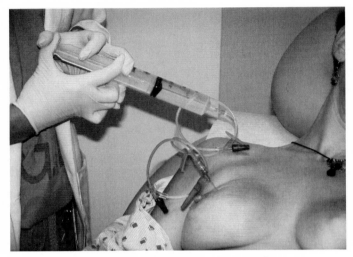

The injection of saline into the expanders

Amazingly, the new bump looked more like a breast! I could feel the skin and muscle stretch; it wasn't really painful as much as it just felt stretched. The practitioner wrapped me in a six-inch wide roll of ace bandage to keep everything in place. I was to wear this until otherwise instructed. I got a spare so I could have one when I washed the other. As I donned my blouse, I looked in the mirror. I now had some semblance of a bust again. Nice!

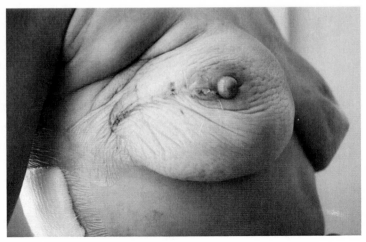

After my first fill without clothes

All in all, it was a pretty full day. As we drove home, I felt myself smirking as though I had a little secret. All I could think of was that jingle from Chili's from a few years ago, Tracy style: "I got my boobies back boobies back, boobies back . . . ." (to the tune of, "I want my baby back baby back baby back ribs"). Although it wasn't much to speak of, I had a little cleavage again! I never purposefully brought attention to my cleavage in the past, but I was so excited to have a little (yes, "little" being the operative word!), that I found myself having some fun with it, saying things like, "So, what do you think of my new rack?" to a selected few. These bumps clearly fell into the category of "sporty," but I was very pleased and happy because it felt as though I was moving in the right direction. I just wanted my body and life back to normal . . . whatever that may be!

Back at the homestead, the kids had returned home after being over at their dad's for his long weekend. It was nice to have them back. It was also nice to come home from appointments to find that the "dinner angels" left dinner in a cooler on the front stoop. Although I love to cook, the meals were such a blessing.

I had a day on the soccer field with Don. I still couldn't drive (that would have to wait until the next Wednesday, when I would go back to have my last two drains taken out), so Brian dropped me off at 3 pm and picked me up at 5. It was awesome being out with the middle-school boys' soccer team. I had signed up to coach their team this season but had to step down, but I still tried to be there when I could. Just those two hours outside took a lot out of me. The parents of the boys stepped up and made this easy for me. We all live by the saying, "It takes a village." My village peeps had my back.

The next day, I went back to work for the morning, and then ran a number of errands and attended Samantha and Donald's soccer games. It may not have been a lot to do before surgery, but it was a lot now. I heard my body loud and clear, and it said, "Only one big thing a day, please." That meant work OR a game, OR an outing. Not two, not three, but one of those things. I knew if I *had* to, I could get through it . . . but that day left me exhausted and hurting, and it took a day or two to recover, and that was no fun. So, I decided to tackle one thing a day, and I relied on the village for the rest. Onward, Outward, and Upward.

CHAPTER FIVE

Pretending Things Are Normal

Saturday, October 1, 2011

I HAD A very busy week, but not in the busy way that was familiar to me in the past. Doctors' appointments, prioritizing what my "one big thing" of the day would be, and trying to manage things indirectly, without being in total control – that's what my life was filled with now. This (temporary) change in lifestyle was exhausting and frustrating.

I was able to get to Donald's first win at his soccer game. I was true to my "one big thing," including helping with soccer, but I was also able to help out a few times when I had the energy to do so. Don's coach was totally supportive of my day-to-day life and seemed to appreciate my help when I could offer it on the field. I got outside in the beautiful fall weather and exercised my lungs. (Those who know me know that I "have a set of lungs," even after my bilateral mastectomy!) The boys could hear my suggestions and instructions for sure!

The girls were busy and working hard. The day-to-day grind continued. We all tried to keep things as normal as could be. It is beautiful how children force life to go on. They still asked, "What's for dinner and when will it be ready?" They still declared at the eleventh hour that their sports uniforms were dirty or nowhere to be found. They still texted and said, "I need a ride home," just as I sat down and thought it would be a good time for a nap. They still threw things out like, "Can we have a Halloween party before you start your chemo?" They still said, "Mom, I'd like to start up gymnastics again; I really miss it." They still asked for me to be there on college tours. Thank God for these distractions. They made me feel normal . . . and exhausted. Yet, I wouldn't trade it for anything.

As I mentioned, I aimed to accomplish one big thing a day. Sometimes two. I made a list of seven things, and typically, only three got done. It was frustrating. I simply ran out of juice. I still hit a wall at around 2 pm, when I needed to sit down and take a load off. I also realized that when I got short with the people who cared for me and loved me, it was my body telling me that I needed to take something for pain. I tend not to acknowledge pain, but my body let me know in other ways that it was there and needed to be tended to. It took a while to recognize this signal, but once I figured it out, I was grateful that I understood what was going on so I could fix it.

I held a meeting for work on Wednesday morning from 7:30 am to 9 am. The attendance was good, and I was very pleased with how things went. Brian drove me to and from that, and then down to Boston that day because I still wasn't supposed to be driving. It felt good to be productive with a rather upbeat and seamless meeting. On Friday, I worked at the Coumadin Clinic and saw patients from 9 am to noon. THAT felt GREAT! Doing what was normal and what felt familiar really helped me. Although I didn't mind at all talking about what was happening to me with this diagnosis, remembering what it was like to live life Before Cancer and feeling those glimpses of normalcy recharged my batteries.

I was in contact with the local cancer center and set up an appointment for the coming Friday (October 7) to meet with an oncologist and have my consultation. We would then set things up for the following week so I could actually start chemo. I would have to work with the center to coordinate a date, but starting the week of the 10th would put me at five weeks after surgery. I was feeling strong and ready.

I signed up to walk with the "Bear Boobies," a group that was assembled for the Cancer Walk in Concord. It was comprised of moms of the girls' varsity soccer team but allowed anyone willing and able to walk. Just in case my chemo treatment started the days right before that, I asked Abbie to be my proxy. I tried to do my part by getting sponsors and donations.

When I look at the amount of money raised for breast cancer, I am astounded. Being a patient, I am grateful for the state-of-the-art technology that allowed my cancer to be found and treated so quickly. However, if it were up to me, I would use some of this money to make a post-op bra that isn't so barbaric. I mean, really, is it too much to ask to get one that is both functional and has a little "bling" or pizzazz? The bras they gave me post-op were SO utilitarian and ugly, and how is a woman to feel beautiful with such a hideous thing? I would be sure to put in my request that at least some cancer research money go toward the development of a "Bra-Dazzle" kit to spice up the bra.

I continued to travel to Boston for my post-op checks with my plastic surgeon once a week and these appointments fell on Mondays. One week, due to the practitioner's schedules, my appointment fell on a Wednesday. And naturally, Monday was when all of the questions started to pile up, making Wednesday feel a lifetime away. *Is the swelling under my arm normal? When will I be off of these pain meds? And where can I find a wire brush so that I can sufficiently scratch these areas around my drains? The itching is driving me mad!*

Wednesday came, and I FINALLY got the last two drains pulled! (Praise God!) I had initially affectionately referred to them as "bobbles" but realized quickly that I actually had little to NO affection for them, and henceforth started referring to them as "the f'n drains." (That's the G-rated version.) I was HOPING that after two weeks, I'd have them pulled (as I was under the impression that I wasn't allowed to drive until then). But up until this past week, fluid kept draining in the remaining ones and there was too much daily output to have them all pulled, so I lived with them yet another week. They were more than just a "thorn in my side." If I moved the wrong way, it felt as if someone were taking a pair of needle-nose pliers, pinching, then twisting the skin on my side where they were sutured in. Then there was the fun of trying to find a comfortable position to sleep each night. Although I safety-pinned them to my nightshirt or undies so they wouldn't get tangled, I was always fearful that I'd inadvertently pull them as I rolled over in my sleep. I wince just thinking about it.

One of my biggest challenges was to figure out how to hide the drains when I went out, so innocent children passing by didn't see them and run screaming for their mothers. There weren't too many options. When I was home, the easiest option was to pin them to the outside of my waistband, which made Don uncomfortable, because there they were in plain sight, serous drainage and all. (Ew.) The other option was that I could pin them inside my shirt somewhere around my waist, where it ultimately looked as if I had an inner tube under my shirt or an advanced case of "muffin top" (not the look I was aiming for, mind you). What seemed to be the best option for outings was to just tuck them into the back of the waistband of my pants, which worked the best, except when riding in the car. Anyway, those suckers couldn't have been pulled fast enough.

When I first learned about my diagnosis, I made the conscious decision NOT to look at long-term statistics for recurrence and outcomes of "five-year survival rates." I figured none of these statistics included ME, and many are from years ago that are only now being published. Since then, haven't we made leaps and bounds in treatment? So, why worry myself with such information? (Unless the numbers are good, then bring them on!) My philosophy was *ignorance + optimism = bliss.*

So, when I went to the original plastic surgery consult, the burning question of, "How will I look when everything has been completed?" was at the forefront of my mind. I'd hoped to perhaps see pictures of what things would look like – before and after – just to get a ballpark idea. The plastic surgeon never offered me any pictures to look at, yet when I was leaving, I saw a huge photo book in the hallway. Shannon, who had accompanied me to the appointment, reinforced my thoughts. "You should look if you are curious. Now is the time. We're here, and you need to have all of your questions answered." I waxed and waned and ultimately decided that it might make me more uncomfortable. Seeing those pictures of other women seemed to fall into the same mindset of hearing five-year survival outcomes. Those pictures may be there (of women in similar situations) to demonstrate the work of the plastic surgeons, but they were not me, and I wouldn't look like them. And most importantly, I didn't know their stories. What kind of breast cancer did they have? Were they in perfect health and did they have perfectly sculptured runners bodies? Or were they smokers with other complicating comorbidities? Were there extenuating circumstances to their treatment? Because I didn't know, I decided against looking. I didn't want to see a great outcome and set my standards too high, only to realize that the unknown decapitated breast picture belonged to a person who had a totally different set of circumstances. If I ended up with some sort of complication and it didn't turn out like the picture, I didn't want the disappointment. (Plan for the worst, hope for the best.) But walking away left me feeling that I still didn't *know* what to expect, and I had to rely on faith and acceptance that things would work out.

Now that the drains were all out, the other reason for seeing my plastic surgeon was to continue to receive my weekly fill. At this visit, I asked the ARNP how they would know how many cc to inject. She told me they would work with me to see how full to make me. The weird part was, she didn't know me prior to surgery. So, she didn't know, other than observing how my body tolerated the fills, what I looked like or what I was expecting. Medically, I had to trust her. But from a self-perception standpoint, she had to trust me, because only I would know when I felt like me. I found that even though I was just starting, every fill gradually made me feel more like me.

I also learned at this visit that the Tegaderm (a clear, water-resistant dressing) that covered the incisions on the lateral sides of my breasts, would remain for four weeks post-op. So, until it was removed, the overall orientation of my breasts seemed different. As grateful as I was to keep my nipples, they each had their own agenda . . . one looking west, the other looking east. I had a breast version of Marty Feldman eyes. (For those who don't know who Marty Feldman is, Google an image of him. That'll sum it up for you.) No offense to Mr. Feldman, but that is not my idea of sexy. Sigh. *This is temporary, this is temporary, this is temporary.* That is the image I will leave you with until next time. You're welcome.

CHAPTER SIX

The Breast Case Scenario

Monday, October 10, 2011

THIS WEEK WAS a big one for me, because not only did I get a fill in Boston on Monday, I got to meet my *local* oncologist on Friday. I was extremely nervous for this visit. I wasn't fearful that I wouldn't like her or the local facility, but I was in knots worrying that when I got there, she would break unexpected bad news to me that I didn't see coming. I like to have all of the facts so I can formulate a plan. My medical oncologist in Boston had prepared me well for my next steps. But what if I got to this cancer center and the oncologist there said, "I reviewed your bone scan, and I saw something suspicious, and we want to hold off treatment and do further testing to find out what it is"? The thought of that was paralyzing. What would I do then?

This is the fear that anyone diagnosed with cancer faces every time there is a new scan, test, or follow up. And dealing with it is all consuming. I found myself always preparing for "the other shoe to fall" and then trying to picture how I would handle it. It's exhausting and scary. The diagnosis of cancer alone blindsided me, so I knew I wasn't immune to unwelcome news. Some people suggested that I take things "one day at a time." It truly was one *breath* at a time, and some days, even one heartbeat at a time.

This fear was distracting and frustrating, because all of this worry overrode my much-needed positive energy, which I needed so I could think about important things like: *What outfit would I wear to my first chemo appointment? Does one dress casual and comfortable or go in with a bit of flair? Capris? Jeans? Is this a leg-shaving event?* Was it ironic that I would think of that because within three weeks I wouldn't have any hair? The best advice came from my friend Goat (his nickname), who recommended that I don a pair of "pretty shoes and kick ass." *Why didn't I think of that? What shoes* will *I don that day to kick ass? My Vegas "Steel-Toed Heels" seem appropriate, right? What will I have for breakfast and bring for lunch?*

Although I'd been told nausea and vomiting are rare due to the pre-chemo "cocktail" I'd be given, I felt compelled to consider what the foods that went *down* would be like *coming back up* – just in case. When I was a kid, I got sick once after eating Spaghetti-O's. (Sorry, graphic visual there.) So as a result, I was thinking that my breakfast choice should be something flavorful but perhaps not so "red."

More thoughts I had: *What things will I bring with me to kill the time as the poison-that-is-my-friend runs into my veins? Books, crocheting, computer, guitar? Maybe now is the time to write some clever yet meaningful lyrics to a song like, "I've Got the Alopecia Blues."* I needed my energy for answering such questions. It is such a shame when energy is wasted on worry.

But regardless of trying to keep it at bay, worry seemed to prevail early in the week. The good news was that Friday's appointment allayed all of my fears about being blindsided with bad news, and it did turn out to be the "breast" case scenario.

Being in the healthcare industry, I know how it feels to run behind schedule and have patients waiting for you. I work part time in a Coumadin Clinic managing patients on blood thinners, and I always hope that the time I take with patients doesn't leave them feeling rushed (which never seems to leave a good impression). I want to know that I have adequately answered their questions so that when we're finished, their experience has been positive, they're at ease, they're informed, and, dare I say, they might have even enjoyed it? I bring this up because when it's my turn to wait as the patient, I'm of the mindset that it will be worth the wait because great providers are a blessing and will take whatever time is needed so that I won't get the bum's rush out the door.

My theory proved true that Friday morning – my new oncologist was running late, but it was a true blessing. When it was my turn, I wasn't rushed at all. In fact, I felt as if I were her only patient and had all of the time in the world to ask and understand everything she had to review with me. She made me laugh a number of times as she reviewed my history. First, she asked if I were a smoker (only a little out my ears when I am irritated). Then she said, "This one always confuses me. It says here that you're a 'social' drinker, but I'm Irish, and I have no idea what that really means!" It was like talking with a friend.

I especially liked her when she told me during my physical exam that my expanders and plastic surgery looked great *already*. It was nice to hear such positive unsolicited feedback from a healthcare professional. Her comments were real, though, as she iterated that my upcoming treatment would not be "easy." She said there should be giant pins that say, "I'm going through cancer treatment," so that people around me could understand my behavior or know that I was going through challenging times. I addressed how a bald head might also act as a giant pin, and we both agreed: It does.

She prepared me for fatigue and described it very realistically as similar to when you stay up way too late at night and then have to get up again only after a few hours of sleep. You CAN push through, but you feel exhausted by the end of the day. The first four doses would be given every other week, and I would have good and not-so-good days, but she never described it as unbearable. Frankly, if it was, I'd rather go in with the positive things in mind and not know. Tolerance to treatment is very individual. I would find my own way.

I hated to start the next Thursday, because it was Samantha's eighteenth birthday. We had celebrated with a dinner the previous Sunday, and she would get her traditional breakfast in bed on her actual birthday. The timing stank, but I needed to get this party started. I was essentially cancer free. They removed the tumor and the cancerous lymph nodes surgically. Done. However, there were rogue cells looking for their moment to jump on the bloodstream railway and jump off in an unwelcome and unfamiliar station. My friend Frieda told me that we should get going "before one of those cells notices that no one is guarding that train." I agreed.

I was told that before we started, I would need an echocardiogram, because one of the side effects of the first treatment of chemo is heart failure. Awesome. Although I was well within the "safe dosing" end of the spectrum, they needed to be sure my ticker was OK, and this would give them a baseline. I would have pre-chemo labs drawn and an appointment with a nurse on Wednesday. The nurse would go over chemo-related things such as, for a day after treatment, flush the toilet twice if you have animals (in case they are dumb enough to drink from the toilet), because there are toxins excreted in urine. Who knew? If Garwood (my black lab) could eat and subsequently poop out an athletic sock and not die, I should think he'd breeze right through a few little namby-pamby "excreted toxins." Maybe he would glow in the dark when we let him out at night? Anyway, the nurse would review everything so that I'd be prepared and all questions would be answered prior to showing up.

I was given a "tour" of the treatment area. There was a snack station, and I could order lunch at the hospital if I wanted. There was Wi-Fi so I could bring my computer, there were TVs with DVD players and head phones, there were warmed blankets, and there were people who came around to do Reiki as well as hand and foot massages! I know, it sounds like a slice of heaven, and you are all so envious.

The Cancer Walk would be on Sunday. It wasn't great timing, because it would be three days after my first treatment, and I didn't know how I would be feeling. But after a story Samantha told me, I wanted to walk it more than ever.

At the end of the previous week, Coe Brown Northwood Academy (my daughters' high school) had an assembly where Coach Hils (Sam's soccer coach and Abbie's teacher) spoke to the student body about the importance of finding a cure for cancer. He said that if each student sacrificed and donated the dollar that they would spend that week on a candy bar, they could raise more than seven hundred dollars. As he stressed the importance of finding a cure, Sam heard a group of boys behind her, talking throughout most of the coach's speech. Then, she overheard one boy say, "No hair? No boobs? What's the point?"

It left a pit in my stomach. When she told me, I could only imagine how hurt and infuriated she felt. All I could do was shake my head and pray that those boys don't ever have to be in her shoes one day. They clearly didn't realize that they had a peer as close as a row in front of them who was worrying about her mother's immediate and distant future and how scary that was.

What these boys failed to see is that besides the anxiety of an uncertain future and the physical side effects of treatment, a woman going through treatment is also battling how to *feel like a woman* with absent or altered "boobs" and no hair. Well, I was, anyway. I didn't even know how to muster the energy to deal with the judgment and ridiculous conclusion that I would not be "worthy" without either of those two things. Perhaps we could simply chalk it up to a comment made from an awkward teenage boy who was trying to be funny at an uncomfortable moment because the word "breast" was being used during an assembly. I'm sure there are numerous other reasons why those dumb words could have been uttered – I can't claim to understand the minds of these teens. Regardless of the off-color remark, what I walked away with was how moved I was (and continue to be) that teachers, coaches, and students were trying to make a difference, perhaps with me in mind. It made me want to walk that "Making Strides" walk even more.

So, medically speaking, the week would be busy. I'd be in Boston for a fill on Tuesday, schedule an echo sometime before Thursday morning, get labs done, go for a nurse's visit, and then finally have chemo on Thursday. It's funny how my one big appointment a week used to be my trip to Boston. Now, the fills were old hat and routine, and I was comfortable with them (not to mention excited to see the "progress!"). Going forward, chemotherapy would be my new "big" appointment to contend with. And I would make the breast of it.

CHAPTER SEVEN

My First Chemo Treatment

Friday, October 14, 2011

HAVE YOU EVER played a game with an opponent whose strengths you didn't know but thought, "I don't know exactly how good *you* are, but you don't know how good I am, either, so bring it on and know that you are in for a challenge"? And that in spite of the odds, you played anyway? That was me on my first day of chemotherapy. Even though I knew it had a job to do, even though I knew I needed it and it wasn't an option, even though I knew chemotherapy comes with some not-so-nice characteristics and is known for playing dirty, I was about to take on two unknown opponents: Adriamycin and Cytoxin.

After starting my day making Samantha's birthday breakfast (belgian pumpkin waffles & Taylor Ham) and serving it to her in bed, seeing Abbie off, and getting Donald to the bus stop, Brian and I headed to the cancer center for an 8 am start to my first day of treatment.

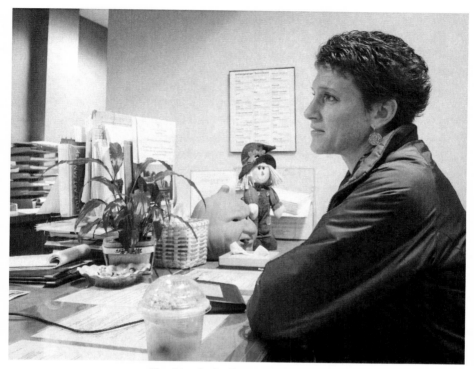

Checking in for Day one of Chemo

The thing I already liked about the cancer center was that it's small enough so that, much like the sitcom *Cheers*, after one day, everybody knows your name. The staff made a concerted effort to make everyone feel welcome. After registration, I was weighed (chemo would be dosed based on a calculation of my height and weight, and yes, I took off my four-inch heels – they didn't count) and we were ushered into Bay 7. I was given a warm blanket and a glass of juice. My nurse, Olivia, came over and introduced herself, and since it was our first visit, told us about what to expect. First, they would double check the doctor's orders and review my lab work to ensure that it was all within normal parameters. If it all looked good, she would then put in the pharmacy request and they would mix up my medications. Olivia did a quick nursing assessment and asked about my current pain and fatigue levels to get a baseline.

Sometimes, when things were going well and I felt normal, I forgot for a minute that I had all of this unknown ahead of me. I didn't *really* feel that all of this was real . . . until the IV went in. The rush of that fluid, always cooler than my own blood, represented a submission of sorts. It was the portal into which poison in a bag was transported into my bloodstream. It was the beginning of a new phase where, yet again, I was not in control. It was the ball and chain for the next few hours. It was uncomfortable; maybe more so mentally than physically. I could exercise, hydrate, take vitamins, pray, and laugh – do everything in my power to try to get better on my own. But the reality of the IV said to me, "As much as you're doing, it's just not quite enough. Step aside; the medicine needs to take over now." Once the IV was in, I had to succumb. I could no longer deal with it MY way; I had to deal with it according to a medical protocol. It was the same thing that made my surgery real. Now, it made the reality of chemo undeniable. It was temporary, but it symbolized something that I could not do for myself: rid my body of any cancer cells that might be lurking in the shadows. As Olivia found a great vein and started my IV without effort, I experienced the taste of salt in my mouth for a few seconds, a weird side effect of the normal saline flush/ fluids. It was time to relax and let the medicine do its thing.

Shortly after, my oncologist came in to meet with me, check me over, and make sure all questions were answered before things got officially started. As before, she was upbeat and comforting and didn't leave until all questions were answered. She promised to swing in again.

Brian stepped out to do some errands while the pre-meds went in. There were four: an anti-emetic (medicine to stop vomiting) to block the receptors in my brain that might think it would be a good idea for me to vomit, another that worked similarly, a med to help stop other gastric issues, and a steroid to help prevent an allergic reaction (that would suck). As these were going in one after the next, Diane, a woman who had given me Reiki before my biopsy back in August, stopped in. She offered hand or foot massage, aromatherapy, or Reiki. I am a sucker for a foot massage, so this was a no brainer for me. During the whole administration of the pre-meds, she rubbed my feet, and we talked. (She taught me a little about reflexology in the foot and aromatherapy.) I was so relaxed and comfortable that I think I almost proposed to her . . . I was just a little lost in the post-massage euphoria. Either that, or it was the pre-meds.

Next on the pre-chemo event schedule came the pet therapy. A little springer spaniel named Titan, with eyelashes *an inch* long (I kid you not!) was brought in to make her rounds. She sat complacently in her owner's arms as she conceded to ear rubs and head pats. She was so soft and clean . . . and calm. I pictured Garwood, my eighty-five-pound black lab, in that role. As sweet as he is, for starters, his breath could "knock a buzzard off of a shit wagon." So, for those with queasy stomachs, I'm not sure if the strongest anti-emetics would even work. There's that and the fact that he *thinks* he's a lap dog, and he's so excitable that I could envision any sort of therapy session with him ending in knocked-over drinks, upturned IV poles, and blood pressure cuffs flying into furniture with the exuberance of his excited tail. Some dogs are meant for pet therapy. Titan is one. Garwood? Not so much.

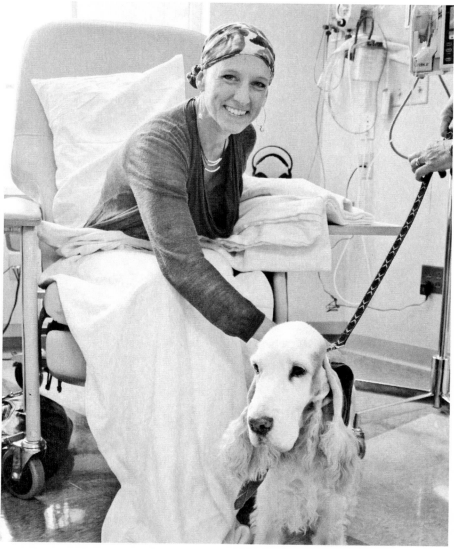

Although this picture wasn't taken until my third round of chemo, I had to include a
picture of this sweet canine!

Pet therapy ended the entertainment, although I kept an eye out for the
Flying Yolanda Sisters or something, but it must've been their day off.

Brian returned just in time for the chemo to start. The Adriamycin was first.
It was an IV push, meaning that the nurse slowly pushed it via syringe for fifteen
minutes. It was bright Kool-Aid red. I wondered how I would feel, knowing

that toxic chemicals were being put into my bloodstream; would it wig me out psychologically?

Olivia explained the strict protocol for the administration of the Adriamycin. It was vital that the Adriamycin be pushed slowly after verification that the IV was still in the vein, because if it infiltrated and went into my tissue, the result would be tissue necrosis, aka gangrene. So, suddenly, I really *wanted* that toxin in my blood and NOT in my tissues!

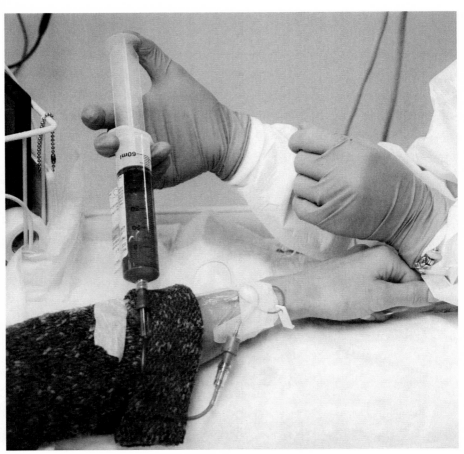

Injection of Adriamyacin

They had a comforting safeguarding system to ensure that the IV was where it was supposed to be. The IV line had a port, where the nurse inserted a syringe and then pulled back on the plunger. When a "flashback" occurred, which was the blood that came back up through the IV *from* my vein, she KNEW she was still in a vein. If nothing came back, there may be a problem. So, the routine was that she drew back (aspirated) and verified the placement with the flashback, then injected a few cc of Adriamycin, stopped, opened the normal saline IV line, and waited for the saline fluids to clear the line. The saline pushed the last of the red Adriamycin gradually into my vein, and eventually the IV line became clear again. They did this because they didn't want to mistake the drug for flashback, since both the blood and the chemo are red. Before administering the next dose, the nurse has to verify placement again – and every time after that until its done.

This was effectively comforting for the first half of the treatment . . . until suddenly, there was no nice flashback. I had a very small gauge IV, and most likely, the beveled end had just rested up against my vein wall, so it didn't allow any blood to flash back. But, before I had time to panic, I was given an extra bolus of fluid to see if it would accumulate in the tissue around my IV site. We didn't notice any. I could also smell and taste the salt in my mouth after the normal saline flush, which was a good sign that the IV was still in my vein. We were finally able to see just a slight return of blood in order to finish administering the remaining dose. I was so glad it went without incident!

The second drug was a piece of cake. It took only an hour. The biggest issue was a non-medical one, where we couldn't get the DVD player to work with the overhead TV. (We had both brought our computers but thought it would be easier to watch a movie overhead.) At one point, four nurses tried to get it figured out as we sat there feeling sheepish and guilty for commanding so much attention. The staff aimed to please in all aspects of the treatment experience, and even though we told them not to worry about it, that it wasn't that important, they were determined to fix it.

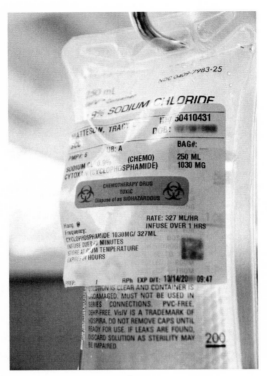

Bag of cytoxin

The next thing we knew, there were only twenty minutes left on the IV. When the alarm went off, that was it. The nurses came, flushed the line, and removed the IV. They gave a few farewell pieces of advice (don't forget to flush the toilet twice; if you have any nausea, don't wait, take a pill right away and be gentle with yourself; don't push it this weekend), and we were off to schedule the next infusion. Done. And not one wave of nausea or lost hair.

I had slight nausea on the first evening of my first chemo, so, as instructed, with the first inkling of queasiness, I popped a Compazine. Maybe it was just nerves, but I didn't know if the nausea would pass or get worse, and I didn't want to take that chance. I hate vomiting.

My sister and Shannon both visited. I felt surprisingly well. Regardless, the nausea (a two on a scale of one to ten) totally abated when Brian gave me Reiki that night before bed.

Yet, I was restless that night and didn't sleep particularly well. Perhaps it was due to wondering if I would feel differently when I woke up, or having to pee (red pee!) from all the IV fluids, or maybe it was the dream that the IV push of the Adriamycin infiltrated into my arm and looked like a marble under my skin. I woke up holding my arm. Nothing prepares you for the mind spins, as unrealistic as they are.

I had thought I'd be giving myself the subcutaneous injection twenty-four to forty-eight hours after chemo to keep my white count up, but as it turned out, it had to be done at the hospital. I thought that was kind of dumb when I could just do it myself, but then I found out that the injection is mucho bucks . . . one person thought it was five thousand dollars; another told us it was eleven thousand. The shot that was injected into my belly could have been a nice down payment on a car! I guess the insurance companies don't trust the common layperson to go home with such an expensive medication. Truth be told, I was relieved not to have to take on such a huge responsibility.

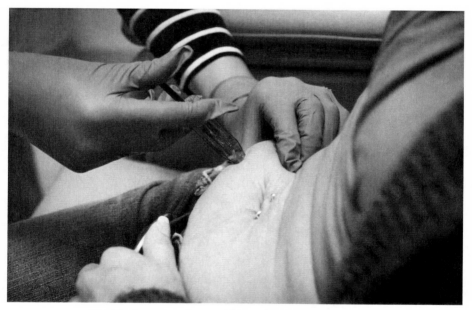

The Neulasta shot that could be a down payment on a car

When I went in for the five-million dollar injection, I was informed that feeling good the day of and the day after chemo was quite normal. It's the following days after the infusion AND the injection that usually get hard. Bummer. But, perhaps a positive attitude would help me glide through the next few days, too. I planned to walk in the cancer walk in Concord that was coming up, and I hoped I could do the entire walk, although as a contingency plan, they did have a "survivor" walk for those not up for the whole thing.

That sums up my first treatment in a nutshell (a rather large and longwinded nutshell). Once the unknown of the next few days passed, I would face the reality of hair loss. This was my next hurdle, and it was right around the corner.

I knew I would lose my hair. It was a gimmie. But I had been doing a lot of thinking about how I would handle it. Yet again, I found a similarity between pregnancy and cancer treatments, only this time in an "it-turns-your-body/life-upside-down" sort of way. As a first-time expectant mom, I had no way to know how it would really feel or how I would handle my delivery. You can put a birthing plan together: build your playlist of soothing music, bring the yoga ball, practice your deep breathing, whatever. But often, when the big day comes, your soothing music irritates the crap out of you because you're trying to deal with this excruciating level of pain, and your partner stands at your side thinking, "Holy crap, what was I supposed to do with this ball, and which one of us is supposed to be breathing?" Even with the best of intentions, a well thought-out plan can come unraveled in the blink of an eye, or, more accurately, the release of a hair follicle. Hair loss, like a delivery, *will* come. I knew it would happen, and I knew I would be bald. I accepted that it would be a matter of time, and although I thought I would handle it OK (like a birthing plan), I didn't know how it would really turn out, physically or emotionally.

The nurse told me that some people say it hurts when the hair follicles "release," yet others don't feel it at all. They just see these clumps everywhere they go – on their pillow, in the shower, on the floor, on their clothes. The bottom line is, you can hide the fact that you were diagnosed with cancer until you are bald. Then, this telltale sign might as well be accompanied by a flashing neon sign that says, "CHEMO PATIENT." Although many medical diagnoses are kept fairly quiet and are so personal, this one isn't. There is simply no denying it. Of course, I wasn't trying to deny it; instead, I was trying to anticipate how I would feel when "Tracy Meets Alopecia." As I saw it, there were two ways this could go down.

The first: I could watch my hair come out in chunks. I wasn't wild about that thought at all; it felt as if it would be a painstakingly cruel reminder of a lack of control. It's the reference I made earlier about playing an opponent you could know only a little about. Letting my hair fall out would be when "Alopecia" got control and pulled out the stops and said, "HA! TAKE THAT!" Alopecia: 1, Tracy: 0. Would I walk away from that round thinking, "Well *that* sucked," or would I take pre-emptive actions and just shave it BEFORE that all started?

In the second scenario, I would take control. *Yep, I like the sound of this already.* I called my friend/hairdresser, whom I'd been with for almost ten years. Although my hair was already short, she suggested I get one more trim. Even if all the hair loss happened within the next two weeks, this would make it easier so that when I wanted to shave it, I could easily clip it down to half an inch first, and then we could do the close shave. I wouldn't let Alopecia get the first and only point. The score would be Tracy: 1, Alopecia: 0. In addition, I planned on making it a family event. I didn't want the kids to see me with hair one day, and walk in the next without. We agreed that we'd all do it together. Each kid could take a swipe, shave their initials, and do whatever, before the close shave. No shocks. Everyone included. And documented by Brian.

The other thing I did to feel better prepared was get a couple of caps to keep my head warm and to give my scarves some *gription*. (That's a word I made up.) I also bought a couple of hats and crocheted a couple. One came out goofy . . . pointy at the top, so I tore it out and started over, but the other I liked. It would be an easy one to throw on first thing in the morning or when I was hanging around the house. On the website where I ordered the store-bought caps, there were a plethora of items. False eyelashes (I got some already), Velcro bangs (good Lord), and various types of eyebrows.

I need to give a little shout-out to the unsung follicular heroine of my face: my humble eyebrows. God love them. Low maintenance, but always there, never demanding a bit of attention. As unpretentious as they are, once they were gone, my face would change. But lo and behold, there were a number of options at my fingertips: draw-on crayons used with a brush to make the brows look more like hair, real human hair stick-ons (similar to eyelashes), and even *tattoo eyebrows* that last three to four days. These were all realistic options, but I was no eyebrow pro. What would happen if I put on the tattoo crooked and had to endure the next four days looking perplexed (if one was higher than the other), surprised (if they were both placed too high), or even angry (if placed too low or angled the wrong way)? I was glad there were options, but I needed to see how I would look eyebrowless before I move forward with any of these choices.

Going forward, I would enjoy my appetite, my feeling good, my eyebrows, my eyelashes and hair – good hair day or bad hair day; either way, it would be a "hair day."

Sunday would bring the Cancer Walk; Tuesday, I would have my last haircut (Lord willing) for a while; Thursday morning, I would meet with a holistic oncology doctor who would go over diet, exercise, and the like; Thursday evening, I would go to pick out a wig that my hairdresser/friend Lisa would cut to look like my current style; and Friday, I would go back down to Boston for a fill. I was hoping to breeze through all of it.

CHAPTER EIGHT

Meeting the Master Sergeant

Tuesday, October 18, 2011

WHEN I GRADUATED from nursing school, I was commissioned as an ensign in the US Navy. After taking my nursing boards, I was required to spend a six-week training period to "learn how to be an officer." I had heard that this was just a formality where nurses and lawyers were sent to "fork-and-knife school" in Newport to learn things like rank, who to salute, the Military Code of Justice, and how to correctly wear a uniform. The year I went to Officer Indoctrination School (OIS), however, there was a change in plans. Due to an unusually high number of officers in need of training, a sample group of about eighty of us were sent to Pensacola, Florida, to be trained along with the aviator officer candidates by Marine Corps master and gunnery sergeant drill instructors. I quickly realized that I was not in Kansas anymore, and this was not the "fork-and-knife school" we were promised. This was the real thing.

Immediately, if not sooner, I learned that I was no longer in charge. Charm, control, and sense of humor (among many other things) were checked at the door. If your talent was batting your eyelashes and flashing a convincing smile to get what you wanted, this was seriously the wrong place for you. There were no formal in-person introductions to any of the instructors ahead of time. There was no opportunity to go up and shake hands and smile at the master sergeant and say, "It's very nice to meet you. I look forward to getting to know you over the next two months. Let's take a minute and sit down and chat so I can tell you a little about myself. I like to read, cook, garden, play guitar, laugh, and take long walks on the beach . . . ."

Instead, our introduction consisted of a sobering face-to-face encounter with a man with zero percent body fat, who screamed at us at the top of his lungs. To this day, I could still pick his distinguished, bellowing, and cussing voice out of a crowd. He was in charge. Conversations that used to be normal and polite were now not even a consideration. I couldn't even make eye contact with him. I didn't dare after hearing him scream, "GET YOUR EYEBALLS OFF ME!" at the nurse five feet down the line. This man told us when to get UP (by throwing metal trash cans down the hallway at 0400), when to eat, when to speak, how to dress, how long to shower (three minutes) and how long to run. And yes, this was voluntary – I signed up for this and knew it would only be temporary. The key rules were: don't try to do too much (or you'll stand out and be sorry), don't hold anyone back (or you'll stand out and be sorry), and understand that things will not always go perfectly.

This sounded familiar. Although I didn't hear the voice of Master Sergeant Ryan in my cancer journey, I did see the irony. I got to meet "Master Sergeant Chemo." I went in anticipating that I'd be able to push through at my own pace, thinking I was prepared and as informed as I could be. Over the weekend, however, I realized that like Master Sergeant Ryan, this chemo didn't care that I like to laugh, play guitar, or cook. I had little to no say about what I could eat, what events I would attend, or how I would feel. I'd been sent back to Basic Training.

When I went in on Friday for the five-million-dollar shot, I thought I was doing great. I had a great appetite and great energy, and I was in a great mood . . . until the nurse who gave me my shot very gently hinted that it wasn't usually until a few days after the chemo that any side effects may kick in. I couldn't imagine how I could go from feeling so good to rock bottom in a twenty-four-hour period. So, I tried to appreciate the time I felt good. I ate a huge meal on Friday night and was ready to tackle the weekend.

In the early hours of Saturday morning, I started feeling the effects, but it wasn't what I'd expected. I was restless, achy. I'd been having some trouble getting into a comfortable position with my expanders after my last fill, and I still couldn't lie on my stomach. But in addition to that, this was more of a flu sort of feeling, like the way that your joints ache when you have a fever. I stayed in bed until 9:30 am, which is about two hours later than normal. By that time *every* joint, bone, and muscle ached. And not just a little. I started journaling my symptoms, so that after the next round, I could remember what I felt and when and what I did about it. My doctor suggested that I stick to Tylenol, so I took that fairly regularly for the pain. It helped a little, but I just couldn't get comfortable. I used heat packs on the areas that really hurt. When Brian was near and reached out and rubbed my arm or back, I realized how good it felt to have it rubbed. That helped, but he could only do that for so long.

The other dominating side effect was fatigue. Fatigue is sneaky. It isn't cured by a quick power nap; it isn't feeling as if you got up too early and need to catch up on an hour or two of sleep. It is pure exhaustion. It's "even though I moved the remote when I changed positions, it is waaaayyy at the end of the couch now, and I don't know how I can get to it without exhausting myself." It sounds ridiculous, I know. Couple this overwhelming feeling of fatigue with bone pain, and it's a killer combination. I was expecting that I'd feel tired, and that maybe I would have a little nausea (which I did). I also developed about five mouth sores from the chemo, which limited my intake, and things didn't taste the same. I hadn't expected to drink alcohol, but I had zero desire for it anyway. I couldn't even finish my coffee on Saturday due to the smell, and by Sunday, I had lost the desire for that as well.

I have a pretty high tolerance for pain. I don't often get sick, so when I do, it has to be pretty bad to keep me down. That weekend's side effects made me weary and teary. I knew I had to blast through it, and it didn't really do much good to complain when there was nothing that could be done to fix it. A couple of times, however, for no apparent reason, I found myself in tears, just frustrated, overwhelmed and hurting and not knowing what to do with all of the emotions I was feeling. It was a release, at the very least. The tears didn't last long, but they were cathartic.

The "Making Strides" cancer walk in Concord, NH, would take place on Sunday. I'd worked hard to raise money by sending out requests on Facebook and asking my church family and friends in person for donations. People were very supportive. I went into this week well aware that I was about to have my first treatment. Because everyone handles it differently, I thought I could easily be one of the people who would just sail through the treatment. After all, I had a positive attitude, and I was super-passionate about making a difference for the walk this year. I had so many people who had faith in me, who were reinforcing how strong I was, that I didn't want to let them down.

When I awoke Sunday morning and it hurt to roll over to get out of bed, I knew that the walk would be too much. I knew there would be five thousand people there, and the thought of that alone was overwhelming. Normally, I love being around people. But I was exhausted just thinking about trying to keep a smile on my face when I checked in, waiting with this level of discomfort through the opening ceremony, and then walking the actual five miles. Truth be told, my energy was depleted just walking to the bathroom from the couch and back. Yet I was still torn. I still felt as though I were letting people down. Had my sponsors/donors known that I'd be actively *lying on my couch* instead of *walking* the five miles, maybe they would not have donated. I felt as if I were deceiving everyone who sponsored me. And, worse, I worried that they would think less of me because I couldn't push through for a great cause.

Brian watched my struggle. He knew that I wanted to show everyone that I was strong. Finally, he gently said to me, "The purpose of the cancer walk is to raise money to find a cure. In your case, the way you need to cure yourself is to rest and let your body heal. You have many people walking on your behalf. You can walk next year as a survivor." He was right. Healing after chemo *was* part of *my* cure. I couldn't ignore it. I hoped that people would understand.

So, I made the final decision and called in my "proxies," Abbie and Donald. I let them know they would be walking in my place. My sister, Anneliese, and the three kids all met at my house to go in together. Sam had come down with some sort of sickness, but was still determined to walk for me with her team members. They all headed to the walk together. Once I made the decision not to go, I could relax and rest. I tried to let go of any feelings of guilt. This year, the walk would go on without me.

Late in the afternoon, the kids and Anneliese came home with tee shirts, bracelets, banners (Miss America style, with "Survivor" written on it), and medals. They had embraced every part of the day and brought the event home to me (minus the walking). They had all left at 10:15 that morning, and they didn't get back until around 4:30 pm. Seeing how tired they all were made me realize that I had made the right decision to stay home. They proudly carried my torch, as did others.

On Monday, on a one-to-ten pain scale, my bone pain was down to a three or four (from around an eight), but I still couldn't seem to get out of my own way. I kept up with the Tylenol and couldn't make Donald's soccer game, because by the end of the day, I was overwhelmed with fatigue and devoid of the drive I needed to get out of the house. Every ounce of energy was going towards simply keeping comfortable. I just wanted to curl up on the couch, and I hoped that someone would let my ambition know that that was where I would be patiently awaiting its return.

By Tuesday, my pain was down to a mild ache. I felt much more among the living, now that I had a little more – dare I say it? – energy. I did a little work from my home computer, which made me feel I wasn't totally letting down my employer. I got out of the house, too, because I hadn't been out in almost five days since my shot on Friday. I tried my best to listen to my body and what it needed. Even though up until that weekend I thought I knew what was best for me, I had to submit to the new demands from my body for reasons unfamiliar to me. It was hard to relinquish that control.

Master Sergeant Ryan had my platoon run the Pensacola, Florida, beaches with M-1s for training. I remember trying to call cadence on one beach run – loud, so everyone could hear – and as a result, I was nearly doubled over as I dry heaved in pain and gasped for air. But what I didn't know at that time of struggle was that with this intense preparation, I would be able to run nine miles by the end of my six-week training. So, chemotherapy treatments needed to take control, and I had to let them lead. Like Master Sergeant Ryan, the chemo prepared me for what lay ahead, and although at times I felt somewhat defeated, it made me stronger. Oo-Rah!

CHAPTER NINE

Getting a Little Wiggy

Tuesday, October 25, 2011

For Lisa

I GUESS I have *some* vision . . . . For example, I can look at a swatch of color and picture how it will look in a room. I am able to picture how I want to coordinate my outfit and what accessories will work for me. I am comfortable scanning the ingredients of a recipe and visualizing how it will taste. But what I realize I am *not* so good at is picturing what hair, other than my very own, will look like on me. I found out it's not as glamorous as I once thought.

As it turns out, although insurance won't cover a breast MRI to *rule out* cancer because it isn't medically necessary, once you have it, they actually *do* cover wigs (aka cranial implants) with a doctor's order. Who knew? So, I figured I should at least entertain the thought, right? I might have an occasion where "hair" would be the most appropriate option, like for a work meeting or some sort of special occasion. Although I wasn't really sure how to define an official "hair occasion," I supposed it would be better to have a cranial implant than not. So, I spent some time preparing for an outing by looking at wigs on the internet.

First of all, this may be confidential, so keep it on the down low: Raquel Welch has a side job. I thought she was an actress and model, but evidently, being an icon brought her a new and exciting opportunity as a wig designer! Sassy, sultry, practical . . . you name the mood, she has a wig for it. Naturally, each and every cut looks as if it were made for her. In real life, each and every wig is NOT a natural fit. Trust me here.

Lisa, my good friend and hairdresser, very generously offered to accompany me to a wig shop to help me find a wig that matched my natural color, wave, and style – one that would make me feel most like myself. Once we found the right one, she would cut it to match my current style. This was an offer I couldn't refuse. So, one Monday afternoon, she picked me up, and we headed to Concord.

We parked in front of a discreet little shop and headed in. I looked at the wigs atop the white Styrofoam lady-heads in the window. They said to me, "I may not be the Raquel Welch lid you were looking for, but I could easily qualify as her distant cousin." Huh. I wondered if Phyllis Diller were any relation to Raquel Welch, because that was more along the lines of what I was seeing at first glance. This WAS New Hampshire, after all, not Hollywood. I knew right then I needed to go into this with a sense of humor.

The bells chimed as we walked in, and a friendly woman greeted us. She asked what we were looking for. Lisa stepped right up and told her what we wanted; she has done this before with others in my situation, and I was happy to have her take the lead. We were shown to a private room with a chair in front of a mirror. The nice wig lady brought four different choices and placed them in front of us on the counter. They looked like dead animals, only shinier.

She put the first one on my head, starting at the forehead, and stretched it over the back. *Good Lord Almighty on a Popsicle stick. Was I being punked?* I wanted to burst out laughing. It was the most ridiculous thing I'd ever seen!

The hair was meant to be pliable and malleable. With a little water to crunch it up, it could be molded into various styles. She spritzed and sprayed water and played with the hair to demonstrate its cooperation. But the wig kept riding up. Remember the Coneheads from "Saturday Night Live"? Give them a little light brown hair, and that was what I looked like. Not pretty. NEXT!

This one was too big. The area above the crown of my head was clearly oversized. That, and the fact that it also didn't fit tightly made my head look like a bowling ball with hair. "Strike" two.

The third one, well, it had potential. It fit better, was comfortable, and was a pretty close match to my hair color. It had a little wave in it, and, thus far, looked the most like my own hair. We didn't hate it. The woman went out back to see if there were any that might be even closer to my color.

When she stepped out, we looked at a few posters and at a few wigs on the Styrofoam heads in the room. One wig on the head behind us looked sassy. When the saleswoman came back, Lisa asked, "What about that one?" The saleswoman brought it over and put it on me. We waited with bated breath as she slid it on.

I belted out a snort as I stared at myself in the mirror. I was almost paralyzed in shock. Inside, I screamed, "Get it off me!"

The saleswoman's face remained calm and neutral. "What do you think?" she asked, as she fluffed up the back.

I diplomatically responded the best that I could. "I look sort of like I should be a Whoville character on *The Grinch Who Stole Christmas*." Tracy-Loo-Who? I had bangs that hung in my eyes *and* pointed out toward the sky, and long spiky hair that stood up like the stripe of a skunk down the middle of my head. On the sides of my head, the hair fell flat. Hideous yet hilarious. Clearly not the look I was aiming for.

We decided to go back to the third one. I donned it again, and Lisa walked up to me as though it were her salon, and she pulled pieces out and played with them as if she were going to give it a normal trim. Although it was longer than my hair and it was somewhat crazy, it had the most potential of all of the ones we had considered. If I squinted, it sort of looked like my hair when I first get out of bed. *Sidebar: I am not recommending that the aforementioned "eye squinting method" be the determining factor for narrowing down your final choices if you go out to choose a wig. It just happened to give me the "vision" I needed to make my final choice.*

Lisa and I decided that it was realistic to trim the wig up and make it look close to my hair. I was so thankful she was there to make this feel like a normal everyday event: a foreign quest made familiar by a familiar person. It would have been overwhelming and daunting to go in alone and not want to hurt anyone's feelings. Doing it *with* someone, I could take the time to laugh at how truly awful some wigs looked, and I didn't feel bad about it when we inevitably snickered. It didn't feel serious and stifled. Although it wasn't something I would have chosen to do if I weren't losing my hair, it was a good time, yet another adventure on this crazy journey.

CHAPTER TEN

Hair Today, Gone Tomorrow

Friday, October 28, 2011

I AWOKE WITH my scalp hurting. It felt like when you wear a tight hat too long, and your hair mashes down, and you can't wait to take it off and "tousle" your hair back into place. Or, for those with long hair: when you have your hair back too tight, and you can't wait to take it out of a bun, braid, or ponytail. I got out of bed and went into the bathroom and rubbed my scalp.

I looked down. I had hair all over my hands. I took a shower and kept looking at my hands after I washed my hair. Yep. It wasn't my imagination.

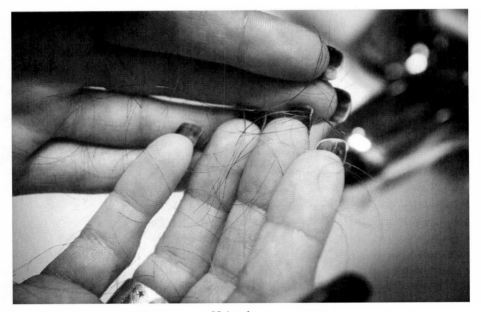

Hair release

I was prepared for it to fall out at about two weeks after my first treatment. I guess I was one of the lucky ones who didn't have to wait the full two weeks.

I made a concerted effort not to touch my hair all day. When I get stressed, I tend to run my hands through my hair, but that day, after I put the gel in it, I didn't dare touch it again. I didn't want to see it fall onto my clothes or computer keyboard.

I knew that I wanted to take action before it started falling out in huge clumps. And I knew it would only get worse from this point on. So, I decided to make the "buzz day" on the following day, after Round Two of chemo. I planned to have Samantha pick up Don; Mom, Abbie, and I would pick up my dad. We called my sister to see if she could make it. Unfortunately, she had to work.

I went to bed that night wondering how bad it would be the next morning. I dreamt about waking up and seeing a "Chewbacca pillow" under my head from all of the hair "release" during the night. In reality, I opened my eyes and found only about a dozen hairs on the pillow.

But when I rubbed my scalp, that's when the big chunks started coming out. In the shower this time, clumps fell out as I washed my hair, to the point that I could see it accumulating in the drain. Hair spread all the way across the tub floor.

On the bright side, my legs and armpits looked pretty darn good.

That morning, my hair gel was like a hair *magnet* to my hands. It was everywhere. It made me feel a little better about the doubts I'd had that maybe shaving it that night would be too soon. But now I knew for sure that it was time. I didn't like how I could put my hand up to a random spot on my head and effortlessly pull out a clump of hair as easily as if it had been casually laid there. As a matter of fact, when I saw Jody at the hospital after my second round of chemo, I joked, "Hey, want a little hair?" and I haphazardly reached up, grabbed a clump and handed it to her . . . totally *not* expecting to find the copious amount that sat in my hand. YIKES! It was really releasing now.

I felt compelled to apologize at that point. "Oh my gosh, I'm so sorry! That was offensive!" Thankfully, Jody has a great sense of humor and was a big support in any and every way I needed her to be, so we just laughed as we stared at the clump. *Good gravy, what am I going to do with this hair now? What's the protocol here? Dropping it on the floor seems not only rude but frankly, pretty darn gross. Where is the nearest wastebasket? Or should I hold onto it until I go outside?* This was another reinforcing moment that it wasn't too soon to shave it off, because, honestly, I didn't want to watch this continue. When I grossed myself out with what I thought would be a harmless gesture of hair sharing, um, I guess that meant enough was enough.

After chemo, we picked up my dad and brought him to my house. Abbie had accompanied me, so she was there with me, and we waited for Sam to pick up Don from school and bring him home.

Meanwhile, back at the ranch, Abbie went upstairs and found my scarves of various shapes and sizes, and we went online and looked up scarf-tying videos to get some ideas of how I could cover my post – hair buzz head. We practiced a number of ties, "rosettes," and braids. There were inspiring videos that made us laugh at their genuineness and others that made us laugh at the ridiculousness.

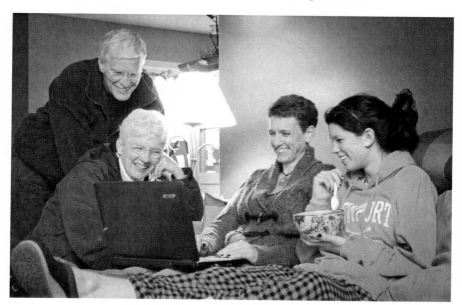

Researching scarf tying online with Abbie, Mom and Dad

Our next job was to get the "buzz room" ready. We opted for the downstairs bathroom. We cleared off the sink so there wouldn't be too much clutter for the pictures Brian would take, put the clippers on the counter, took out the rugs, and placed a chair in the middle of the floor.

It seemed ready, until Abbie said, "It looks like an execution room!"

It did. Only "the chair and the clippers." We opted to put the candle and the Kleenex box back on the counter so it didn't look so ominous. That was much better.

Sam and Don arrived shortly after, and the festivities began.

Since I had cut Don's hair with the same clippers, I thought it would only be fair to let him have the first pass. I'd had the clippers for more than two years before I was told they were supposed to be *oiled* on a regular basis. *Huh, that would explain all of the sudden stops in the middle of a pass across the top of his head . . . and the consequential screaming.* (Come on! I'm a nurse, not a hairdresser . . . although I suppose I could've read the directions.) I told him he could get payback (yes, this time, they *were* oiled and ready).

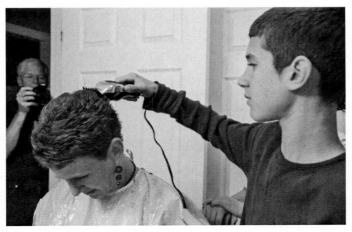

Donald taking the first swipe

We put on a three-eighths-inch guide, and it was anticlimactic. So, we put it down to one-quarter inch, and THAT was the length that showed the cut! Each kid took a turn, after which my mom, dad, and Brian took theirs. Once my whole head was totally shaved down to a quarter-inch long, the kids and my mom took the small trimmers and wrote or drew something into the short cut. Abbie did a breast cancer ribbon, Don made a smiley face, Sam wrote "B-U-ty" (short for beauty but there wasn't enough room for the whole word), and my mom put in a heart. We took pictures to document their heartfelt expressions, then cut all my hair off as close to my head as we could.

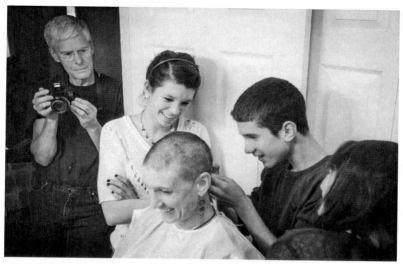

My Dad looking on as Sam, Abbie and Don scribe their special messages

After that, my Dad said that he too wanted to show his support by shaving his head. So, I did the first few swipes and everyone (except Brian, who photographed it) took their turn. It turns out that he and I have very similar shaped heads (who knew?!), and we looked much more alike than ever.

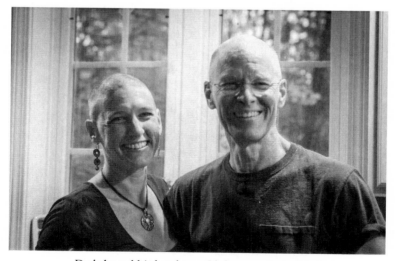

Dad shaved his head too. Oh how we look alike!

That evening was a wonderful bonding experience unlike any other I can think of. Everyone was in good spirits, and we looked forward to doing the cutting together. It didn't take long to get used to the "new norm" of what my dad and I looked like. It didn't seem scary, overwhelming, or weird. If we did it together, I knew that it wouldn't be a shock for the kids to come home one day and see me with no hair. We started off calling it a new tradition, but then decided we really didn't want to have to go through this every year – once in a lifetime is plenty. It was a bonding family event unrivaled by anything we've ever done.

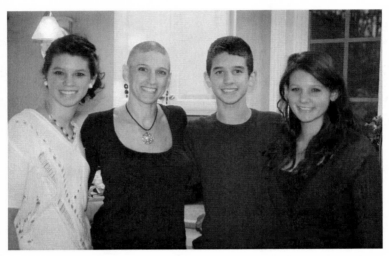

After the buzz with Abbie (left), me, Donald and Samantha

As a show of support, later that week, Donald shaved his head too.

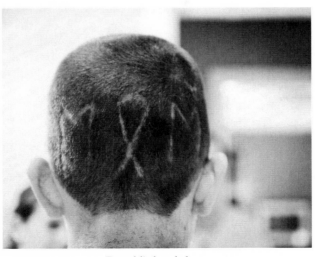

Donald's head shave

CHAPTER ELEVEN

Finding the New Normal

Saturday, November 5, 2011

WHEN YOU START a new job, you have to figure out what is expected of you in every scenario. During orientation, you're introduced to what will happen during a normal day, and you learn how to navigate through it with minimal disruption. Sometimes, under fire, you are thrown into situations where you have to handle the more urgent situations. You then rely on the fact that your experience and knowledge will see you through. You hope that your solid foundation of knowledge will help you efficiently manage the day-to-day tasks and deal with the unexpected.

Although I wasn't sure I was qualified, cancer recovery felt like my new job.

I had to apply a "what's reasonable?" test to my day-to-day life. I was told to "listen to my body" more times than I could count. Before cancer, it was easy to do, because I knew what was normal. If I exercised too hard or too long, or if I did something new, I knew it because I was sore . . . those were my muscles begging for mercy. When I got a cold, I knew it because my nose would be stuffed up. When I was tired from an extremely busy day, I knew I could push through because a reprieve in my schedule was forthcoming, and I'd be able to catch up on rest. My body and I had a good thing going, because it gave me signs that I had gotten to know for years. Recovery from all of this treatment was a game changer.

For example, it was particularly difficult for me after surgery, because the plastic surgeon was the one calling the shots about my activity level. Although I thought I was asking very direct questions about what I could and could not do, it seemed that each time I went in for my weekly fills, I got a slightly different answer. They didn't like to give specific dos and don'ts because "every person is different and everybody reacts differently." As true as that is, that answer made me want to beat my head against a wall. I certainly got it. I *liked* being an individual and knowing that I was healing my own way – unlike, but similar to, the next woman who underwent a bilateral mastectomy. But I have to say, as a person looking for *specific* answers and guidelines, I might as well have been told, "To clarify any further questions, Ms. Matteson, please step into our 'sidewalk entertainment office,' and the mime will clearly outline your restrictions." *Wait, what was that? Did he just mime that I shouldn't vacuum the stairs or that I should stay away from anything with meat in it? I'm not sure; it could go either way.* Like a mime's silent body gestures, surgeons' guidelines can sometimes be equally as vague, leaving much to be interpreted.

Any and all restrictions on lifting, reaching, any sort of exercise, sweeping, vacuuming, resuming sex, starting yoga all got varying answers. I had to realize fully that all suggestions were just guidelines. So, I started asking, "Why?" It helped me to understand the purpose behind the restriction. Some guidelines made sense, like, "We don't want you lifting your hands above your head, because the plastic surgeon had to put in donor tissue to ensure that your expanders stay put and don't shift, and that needs about four to six weeks to heal completely." OK, I could relate to that logic, but I took it a step further and asked what would happen if I overdid it. I was told that if the donor tissue didn't hold everything in place, my boobs could *shift* and end up under my armpits, making my silhouette from the back look like a hammerhead shark from the armpits down. *Oooohhhhhh! Now I was smellin' what they were steppin' in! Why didn't they say that in the first place?!* If the aforementioned "hammerhead shark" theory had been identified early on, it would have been "case closed, nothing further, Your Honor." All post-op protocol would have been followed to a "T." Knowing the consequences was not only helpful, it had a way of driving a point home.

Listening to my body was HARD. I wanted to do – and was used to doing – so much more. Sitting and barking orders was not my forte. But, after surgery, I laid low. I saved my energy for the important things in life, like soccer games and family dinners. I asked for help with rides, meals, cleaning, and shopping. I navigated through activity restrictions, drains, no driving, pain medicines and all that went with that, sleepless nights due to discomfort, weekly fills that changed my body shape. But I eventually regained my strength and started feeling among the living again. I was, in fact, reuniting somewhat with my old body's signs. However, just when I felt I'd gotten a piece of my pre-cancer life back, the rules changed yet again, and chemotherapy began.

During my second round of chemotherapy, I had an altercation with IV infiltration. An uncommon and unfortunate complication developed where, again, I wish I had listened to my body.

When the IV was placed, it was clearly in the vein, because a definite red surge of flashback confirmed that it was good. However, I suspect that when it was placed, the needle accidentally hit the vein internally and left a tiny, undetectable pinhole. That tiny puncture opened just enough to allow the chemo to sneak out of my vein and into the tissue of my hand with the force of the IV push. ADVICE: When the nurses tell you that you will definitely know if your IV isn't in the vein due to the pain and burning, *trust them.* And trust that ANY pain with an IV push is an alert that something is wrong, even when there is adequate flashback. With each push, I watched my hand swell slightly, and the pain made me more and more anxious. Abbie and Mom accompanied me that day, and for their sake, I didn't want to appear weak, whiney, or scared, so I didn't speak up as soon or as forcefully as I should have. I endured the pain of every push until the last one caused me to jump, literally, out of my chair. By then my hand was very red and swollen, so the nurse pulled the IV and placed another one for the Cytoxin.

We elevated my hand and put compresses on it. Just having the IV out helped me, both physically and emotionally. I wished that I had spoken up sooner. I looked at my swollen hand and worried about all of the toxins congregating in its tissue. I had read that Adriamycin was a "vesicant," which is defined as "a drug capable of causing tissue necrosis when discharged from a vessel into surrounding tissue." *Awesome. Did we wait too long to pull the IV? Is the damage done? What should I be watching for? Will my hand turn purple, or black? Are my fingernails going to fall off first? Note to self: Google "how to treat infiltration of a vesicant" when I get home.* Naturally, my nursing brain feared that the gangrene could only be treated by amputation, and I'd go down as a statistic of a breast cancer patient who not only lost her breasts but also a hand due to rare and unfortunate complications.

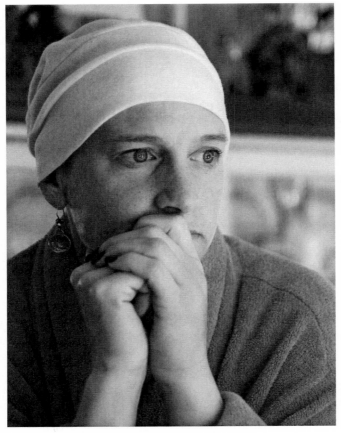

My swollen hand

I'd been keeping a journal of side effects, medications, and activity level since the first day of chemo. I wanted to be able to look back at it after subsequent rounds and say, "OK, that happened, and this is how I handled it." It seemed like a logical plan.

For the first go-around, I documented the bone pain, the level of fatigue, my appetite, my loss of taste for coffee and alcohol, and how everything, even drinks, tasted like a fork. Even though all of the side effects were outlined, I didn't know how rapidly or often they'd come, or what their intensity level would be. I took each and every symptom and labeled it as "expected and normal" or "something to watch." This was going to be my life for the next four months, so I could either choose to try to understand it and put a little rhyme with the reason, or I could let each symptom surprise and therefore worry me. I chose the former.

Clearly, there were too many possible side effects to know every one of them. The big ones stuck out: nausea, constipation, fatigue, to name a few. But it felt like a constant battle to remember which ones to expect.

My oncologist told me that if I got a fever of more than 100.5 degrees, I needed to go directly to the Emergency Room, because an infection could be festering, and I would need blood cultures and IV antibiotics to rule one out. If she said anything with total seriousness, that was it. She reiterated by saying, "DON'T ignore it." That one, I remembered.

After my IV experience, I was hyperaware of any fever symptoms. The tricky part was that as a result of chemo, I experienced menopause symptoms, including hot flashes, which I found to be a lot like a fever. Not to mention that coupled with fatigue and the general bone pain, it ALL felt like a fever, and a person on the anal retentive side might entertain the thought of taking hourly temperatures. No, I'm not that person.

Speaking of conflicting symptoms . . . did I mention that Mother Nature thought she'd shake things up for me and "bless" me with both my period AND hot flashes *at the same* time, just for fun? Evidently, I wasn't experiencing enough superfluous-yet-conflicting symptoms already. Seriously, I didn't know what else was looming around the corner.

At another point, my eyes started burning. *What? A fever, now? Is it a result of the chemo? Is this normal? Is it a hot flash? Or is something else going on?* I had a sore throat and the sniffles, too. *Allergies? Reaction to the meds? A virus?* I took my temperature . . . 100.3 degrees. Crap. Only 0.2 degrees away from upturning my whole night to go sit in the ER to get more needle sticks for the blood cultures and an IV. *Great. When should I panic? I guess not yet. Should I take Tylenol? Or would that be a mistake because it would mask the signs and symptoms of fever and just make things worse?* Sometimes being a nurse worked against me . . . I knew too much, and it stopped me from doing what should be intuitive. I wasn't sure in this case what trumped what.

I opted for sleep, which was the right choice.

Another intense side effect was *fatigue.* It hit at the most inopportune moments and gave me an overwhelming urge to curl up wherever I was, regardless of what I was doing, and close my eyes to "just rest a minute." It hit me after chemo for a few days at a time. By five days post-chemo, it eventually wore off as an all-day thing, and only transient attacks came on. For instance, I was at work writing a letter one day at my desk when it hit. I felt as if I'd need to prop my head up on a pencil to prevent it from dropping down onto the keyboard. I pushed through, because I knew that I had a meeting at noon, and I didn't want keyboard imprints on my forehead. The next time was when I got the urge to dust my living room. I dusted maybe five things, and suddenly, I became UTTERLY overwhelmed. I was on the floor dusting the underside of the coffee table. I thought to myself, "I'm just going to lie down for a second . . . right . . . here . . . ." And I lay down, with my knees up, Swiffer duster draped over my stomach with one hand, the other hand over my chest. I closed my eyes, and there I slept for a half-hour. Fatigue in a nutshell. It's not for wimps.

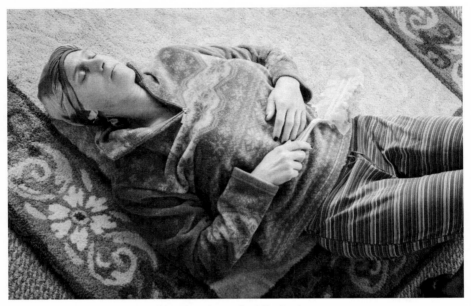

Utterly exhaused while dusting

That brings me to one day's big accomplishment. We (Brian, the kids, and I) unanimously decided that it'd be a good idea to do something as a family outside of the house. I felt somewhat like an anchor holding everyone back from doing anything adventurous, so when everyone was game, I was, too. We decided on an indoor rock-climbing adventure. Enough time had passed since my surgery to allow me to lift and put my hands over my head, so I figured, why not?

It was my first time. I was given a short lesson, and the kids (who had all climbed before) re-familiarized themselves with knots, climbing, and belaying technique. I was filled with nervous energy early on, and I managed to climb all the way up to the top of the wall. (It was a bit scary!) I felt as though I had just conquered Mt. Kilimanjaro! However, I could feel muscles pulling and straining that probably shouldn't be further stressed. I guess I did know my body a little bit more than I thought. I knew it was important to stop. So I belayed from then on.

Brian hadn't seen me climb because he had been paired with Abbie, so I wanted to show him I could do it. I found an easy route and started climbing. But by then, I just didn't have the strength in my chest muscles to pull myself up. I surrendered and tried not to feel defeated when I admitted, "I can't." *Darn. I even have to find the new normal with things I've never done before.* Yes, it was embarrassing to admit that I couldn't make it a second time. But I stopped anyway. Later, when I was home and feeling a little sore, I knew I'd made the right decision. Looking back, it was better that I stopped, because it would be even *more* embarrassing to keep going, tear something, and end up looking like a hammerhead shark, right?

CHAPTER TWELVE

Irony

Tuesday, November 15, 2011

A S PART OF my morning routine, I usually started my day by stepping on the scale. On my way to the daily revealing of "the number," I'd streak by the mirror and catch a glimpse of a body still unfamiliar, even to me. A bright white head with the last remnants of rebellious dark stubble hanging on for dear life and breasts that looked as if someone tried to pack two snowballs onto the front side of a snowman to turn him into a snowwoman, complete with lumps, bumps, and asymmetry. I'd step on the scale, then look down to find a florescent blue screen screaming, "IRONY."

So many generous friends brought over meals that I had more of a variety of dinner options to choose from than I'd ever had before. The problem was my desire to eat. I knew, of course, that I had to eat and that I had to keep up my strength, and I was nothing if not compliant. I paid attention to what went in my mouth, balancing vegetables with much-needed protein and always having a drink of cider or juice on hand to stay hydrated. I thought, "If this was the only thing I ate today, would it be a good choice?" I also knew that the IV steroids I was given before each chemo infusion could play tricks on my brain and tell me that I was hungrier and thirstier than I really was. I needed to be careful about what went in my mouth. I'd just heard a story of a woman who gained thirty-five pounds because the only way to stop her nausea was to eat. I'm glad I heard the story, because, like her, I too found that the slight bouts of nausea abated when I ate something. That was a slippery slope.

I fully believed that the scale's numbers would most definitely be down, so I was flabbergasted to see that the number flashing in bright blue at my feet *mocked* me with a number that I hadn't seen since pregnancy. How was that even possible when I hadn't had the desire to eat in more than four days? Seriously, if Sally Struthers saw my intake in the last four days, even SHE would be worried about me. If it weren't for the fact that I hadn't been exercising, it would have been complete irony that I had not shed *a single pound* through this ordeal. Not that I was going for the emaciated look on top of it all, but I guess I had braced myself for dropping a pound or two as I waxed and waned through my treatments. I ate only because I needed to; I had no wine (Seriously! I KNOW!) or frequent snacks, and yet I had not lost one . . . single . . . pound.

Irony has a way of reminding me that God has a sense of humor. For example, shortly after I found out that the chemotherapy I would receive would cause me to lose my hair, I received a mailing from L'Oreal shampoo products, with a sample of shampoo, conditioner, and hair gel. Hmm. My first instinct was to take a before-and-after shot (with and without hair) and send it back to the folks at L'Oreal, thanking them for the opportunity to use their product.

Another moment of irony was when I received a letter from my OB-GYN office telling me it was time for my annual mammogram. The letter went on to say how the office's newest equipment had a greater ability to detect cancer, and I should call to make an appointment at my earliest convenience. *Hmmm, when should I squeeze this in? After my bilateral mastectomy and before my reconstructive surgery? When would be most convenient? And where was this machine when I needed it six months ago?*

The oncology nurse had recommended that the day *of* through two to three days *after* chemo, I should "swish and spit/gargle" with a combination of either warm salt water or baking soda and warm water, four times a day, eight ounces at a time. It was supposed to neutralize the pH in my mouth and help prevent or lessen the intensity of mouth sores. The salty taste alone made me gag, so doing this ranked right up there with enjoying hemorrhoids.

After my last round of chemo, I forgot to do the salt water gargle/swish and spits. I got no mouth sores that time. Ironic?

Wait, there's more. I learned that when a woman goes through menopause, she encounters a hot flash when her ovaries temporarily don't put out any estrogen to balance her individual yin/yang. (OK, I made up the yin/yang part, but it was basically how it was explained to me.) I likened it to a sort of sputtering a car would demonstrate when it was running out of gas. I had regularly been experiencing said hot flashes and actually found myself wondering, at what point would a woman actually self-combust?

Even with all of the flashes that I encountered, my little dutiful ovaries decided that they were not giving up without a fight. So, lo and behold, one minute I was peeling off my head scarf and any superfluous clothing as my ovaries sputtered out of estrogen juice, and the next, they were triumphantly overcoming the odds by producing yet another period! Ta-da! Look at what we can do! And, what's more, the chemotherapy might not necessarily put me into *permanent* menopause; it might only be temporary, and I would get to do it all over again, naturally, in a few years! Yay?

My latest round with my friend Irony was when I got a "twenty-five percent off a new bra" coupon from Victoria's Secret. Normally, I would love this offer. Bras just aren't made to last, and any discount is a good one and shouldn't be ignored. But this time, as I read through the generous offer from Vicky's Secret, I realized it was so wrong for me on so many levels. First, let's start off with, what are the chances that I could even *find* a bra that would fit these robot boobs? Being totally honest, there was nothing "sexy" about my robot rack, unless you considered having a shelf to rest your dinner on as sexy. I don't mean to sound ungrateful, and don't get me wrong, I knew (and accepted) that the expanders I had in place were doing their job – they were stretching my pectoral muscles so that the silicone implants would eventually be held in place the way they needed to be. Yet I still could not wrap my head around how foreign they continued to look. Breasts should not have corners or edges (I always say). And yet, edges it was until the following summer, when I could have my final surgery. Until then, layering and various means of focal distraction – *not* a push-up bra – were key.

My other reason as to why this offer was all wrong for me was that the VS trend, in case you haven't noticed, is for their bras to push and accentuate *up* a size or two. This was not a look I particularly needed at this time. If my new "girls" were pushed up or out any further, they wouldn't be boobs, they'd be ears. Not to mention that expanders are rugged. They are solid and built to stay put. Out and at attention (albeit one saluting to the front and the other to the northeast) at all times. If I purchased a bra that did either of those two things – push up and out – I'd argue that it should come with a warning label to caution against strangulation. But that's just me.

I did make light of it. I accepted where I was in my recovery. But I did long for the day where I would have soft curves again, not hard edges. Hard edges don't suit me, in any fashion.

I have mentioned that I kept a journal of side effects of the chemo so that I'd know what to expect the next time around. I'd experienced an IV infiltrate, multiple IV sticks, mouth sores, a metallic taste, nausea, constipation (leading to a godawful hemorrhoid and, consequently, an anal fissure, which had to be the most painful thing I've ever experienced), weepiness, loss of appetite, headaches, fatigue, and bone pain. Yep, there you have it – the glamour and reality of chemotherapy. I could sugar coat it, but that is it in a nutshell.

My third round of chemo itself went well, but the journal I kept proved to be less than helpful. What could've been conceived as a pattern fell short.

Going in (most importantly, for the fashion conscious and inquiring minds), I wore pink, faux-alligator sling-back heels and a matching plum print shirt transformed into a head wrap for my noggin. Who needs a lucky rabbit foot when you have those fashions? Again, I felt great the day of chemo. (I attribute it to the shoe choice.) Perhaps though, I overdid it after my Neulasta injection, because I noticed the bone pain crept in early that evening.

The next day, I awoke in awful pain – every bone, every muscle, every joint hurt. It hurt to turn over, walk, and move from point A to point B. An uncontrollable wave of tears overcame me early on and loomed throughout the day. The overwhelming feeling of being fatigued, coupled with the inability to get comfortable, led me to break down and take pain meds. It was a double Oxycodone day. Although I knew the side effect would be constipation, I opted to take it anyway. It allowed me to rest, fairly pain free . . . or at least drugged me heavily enough to not notice or care about the discomfort. Either way, the pain meds helped me through the day and night. The next two days, I fared better; however, I was still achy and void of energy.

There is a lot to be said about being sick and tired of being sick and tired. The fifth day was supposed to be my turn-around day, according to my previous patterns. I knew I was not ready to face work and a "mom's hectic schedule" again, but I did know that feeling better was only around the corner. At least, I hoped so.

After the complication with the IV at my last round of chemo, we found that my hand was still sore and swollen and had even fewer options for IV access for the remaining five treatments. I spoke with my plastic surgeon, medical oncologist, and the nursing staff at the cancer center, and they all felt it was not unreasonable to consider placing a "port" for the administration of the remaining chemo treatments. The downside was that it would be another "procedure." *Huzzah! I will have yet another random lump on my chest!* But the upside was that having a port would allow me to have labs drawn and all IV medications administered through this one site, and I wouldn't have to endure multiple sticks or the fear and anxiety of another infiltrate. I had an appointment for a consultation with my general surgeon, and I hoped he'd be able to place it before the following Wednesday (the day before Thanksgiving), which would mark my halfway point through chemo. Something to be thankful for.

This would be the first year in many that I hadn't hosted Thanksgiving at my home. It made me a bit sad, because I love everything about it. Everything from the setting of the table with good china and carefully chosen name cards, to the chaos of more dishes than I ever thought I had, to the leftovers, to the feeling I get when friends and family at the table hold hands as we say grace. I was grateful that the cancer center could accommodate the timing of my next round the day before Thanksgiving and the shot the day after, so that I could enjoy and actually taste the turkey and feel well enough to enjoy the company of those around me at my mom and dad's house.

I might have taken a lot of time to criticize all of the challenges I was going through, but as Thanksgiving approached, I knew that I had a lot to be thankful for. I had my eyelashes and eyebrows. I got to keep my nipples! I felt pretty darn good about seventy percent of the time. I had a boyfriend who told me daily that I was beautiful, one who made me his priority and was unselfishly available at every turn. I had friends who would do things for me on the drop of a dime, including bring food, give rides, and call, write, Facebook, or email to say, "I'm thinking of you." I had a forgiving and flexible employer who supported me on the days I was just too tired to work. I was surrounded by a family who could not be more encouraging – cousins who texted and emailed me with uplifting messages, a sister who reached out and offered her only free time to visit or help me clean, a grandmother who called and regularly sent cards of encouragement (and said she'd help me write my first book!), parents who worked their schedules around all of what I had going on to be there for me (to drop off a car, food, a bracelet, or to rub my back when I was hurting), kids who checked in when they were away and helped when they could to make life easier for me. I could go on. The gifts and things I was thankful for SO far outweighed the challenges.

So, there was the ultimate irony of them all: I might have been bald and fatigued while enduring this intense treatment, but I was richly blessed.

CHAPTER THIRTEEN

Thankful for Cancer

Wednesday, November 23, 2011

For Brett

A T THIS TIME of year, over the course of the long Thanksgiving weekend, I inevitably sit down and count my blessings and the things that I'm thankful for. The list for me usually goes on and on.

But this time, I wrestled with one particular item.

Was I thankful for cancer?

Thankful? Was that the right word? I thought a lot about it.

Coming to a conclusion started with a conversation with my dear friend Brett.

Brett and I have many things in common. We both love a Virgo. We both love music (although admittedly, his love goes well beyond mine). We both play guitar and sing (but it is his profession, and, truth be told, comparing my playing to his is like comparing a cubic zirconia to the Hope Diamond). I believe we have like personalities – we like to please, we like to make people smile, and, most of all, we have a similar sense of humor. (We've actually had to be separated during meetings of serious nature, where we'd resort to desperate measures and feed off each other to find a little levity.) We both love life and appreciate those around us.

And we both have cancer.

One day, I had a very poignant conversation with Brett, who was diagnosed with a brain tumor a few months before I got my own diagnosis. After an intensive brain surgery and post-op recovery, his next stage of treatment was to have radiation in the same Boston hospital I went to. This meant a seventy-five minute drive down, a fifteen-minute radiation appointment, and then the same drive back – Monday through Friday, for six-and-a-half weeks. Needless to say, Brett and his wife, Dawn, quickly recognized that this daily commute would be wearing, so Dawn started a website where friends could sign up to drive him down each day to ease the driving commitment. I signed up to be his driver for a month of Mondays. On those Mondays, I'd pack water, fresh fruit, or a nut-and-berry trail mix for snacks, then pick him up and head to Boston.

For me, this time was a gift. When else would I ever have the opportunity to enjoy four hours of talking – or not – about whatever we wanted? It was the chance to find out how he was *really* doing – to listen, learn, and love. One morning on the way down, we talked about how fortunate we both felt to have this time together.

In a world where we busily go about our day-to-day lives, we don't fully realize how many people we interact with, or the power each of those interactions holds. But when cancer hits, the people you unknowingly have an impact on start coming out of the woodwork, literally, from everywhere. Brett said that in a strange way, getting cancer was like being at your own wake, except you're alive to experience it. Cancer becomes the great equalizer. It breaks down barriers and gives people the ability to tell you how they feel about you. It empowers people to take a little bit of time out of a busy schedule to make a meaningful connection. And it helps people slow down and become thankful for what they have, or, perhaps, what they don't have. Instead of lying lifeless in a coffin, you're fortunate enough to be able to experience the genuine emotion of the people who show and tell you that they care, that they love you, and that you have touched their lives. It's a powerful gift.

When these Monday trips took place, I didn't yet know that I too had cancer. I remember being in awe when I heard Brett say that cancer was a blessing. *What? How could cancer do anything but suck?* At that time, I couldn't imagine how anyone could reach down so far within himself to find that level of good in all of the hell he'd been through. That's Brett, though. He has been and continues to be a shining example, a true role model, an inspiration, a "Poster Child" on how to have cancer.

I get it now.

Because of our conversation, I held on, with both hands, to his outlook. I was able to look for each and every one of the gifts I've been given throughout this journey. I was fully aware of all of the people who attended my living cancer wake.

On this particular Thanksgiving, I was thankful for so much. Endless meals. A handmade quilt. Tears of friends when they saw me. An incredible and compassionate team of doctors, nurses, and staff. Comments on journal entries (whether it was in person or through Facebook and Caring Bridge, it meant so much to hear about how people read and enjoyed my updates). Hugs, cards, emails, texts. A quiet hour of playing guitar and singing with friends. A trip to Concord for a wig with a friend who made it not only bearable but fun. Visits during chemo or hospitalization stays. Thought-provoking books. Rich, one-on-one time with friends and family during car rides, waiting time at appointments, and healing time at home. Those were all on my Thankful List, because I learned to embrace that opportunity to talk, listen, learn, and love. I learned to appreciate the time I had with the people in my life. I learned to welcome the small gifts given each day, like health, love, and the ability to hug those I care for.

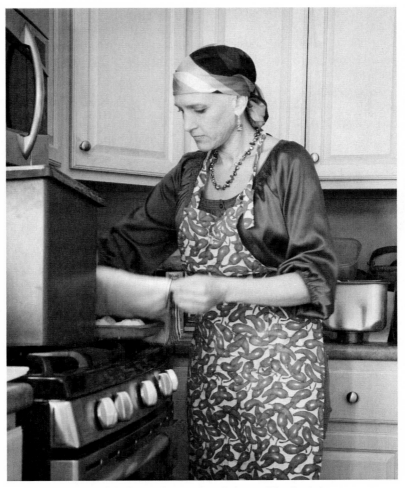

Thankful I felt well enough to bake on Thanksgiving

A lot could happen in the nine-month time frame from when I was diagnosed to when my treatment would end; friends who had babies would have nine-month-olds, Samantha would graduate from high school, Abbie would be driving, and Don would head into his last year of elementary school. The leaves would be back on the trees, the lakes would be filled again, and the loons would be back. Nine months is a long time to put your life on hold and not go out every day with your boots on and make the most of it. I realized that it was also a long time not to appreciate every gift I was given, because, in that time I would have experienced a lot of love, generosity, and support. And although I wasn't in perfect health, it was still clearly a time worth living and embracing.

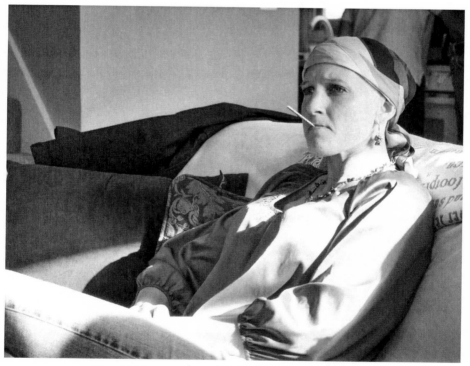

Thankful for no fever and feeling good on Thanksgiving

So, following in Brett's footsteps, I can honestly say that yes, I am thankful, even for cancer.

CHAPTER FOURTEEN

Ode to Chaucer

Sunday, December 4, 2011

Writing entries can get painfully mundane
When describing my journey and every little pain.
In college I loved reading *Canterbury Tales*
So thought I'd try to write in a way that's less stale.

I'll start with good news – chemo's halfway through
I still try to find the bright side with all I do.
I haven't written because there's not much to write
I've been dealing with the BS that goes with this plight.

Thanksgiving was wonderful, I was able to eat
Not one but two meals and two dessert treats.
With my family first then Brian's family at three
I felt blessed with the time and the good energy.

Friday things took a little turn for the worse,
I headed to Dover for my Neulasta shot first.
I had grandiose thoughts of getting lots done
But as the day passed I achieved not a one.

Like picking up salt and shopping for Don
Stopping at work: those options were gone.
As I tried to head out I became winded and found
I had zero energy when my feet hit the ground.

I checked in and Nurse Liv did her spiel
Asking questions about my systems and how did I feel?
The days are gone when all systems are fine
And it feels that all I do is complain and whine.

I had no juice and no appetite still,
This cough lingers on and my hemorrhoid killed,
My bowels seem fine with Miralax's help
My left hand is still red and has quite a welt.

I had a bad dream in the middle of the night
That three doctors had told me I had a new fight,
They said in my lung a new cancer appeared
I cried when I told Liv; it had felt so real.

I headed home to rest and tried not to speak
I couldn't help feeling vulnerable and weak.
I lumped on the couch when the bone pain kicked in
With chills and hot flashes I just couldn't win.

My temperature that evening continued to rise
The 10:30 check was over 100.5.
At 101.2 off to the hospital we sped
When both of us just wanted to go up to bed.

After labs, blood cultures, and a sample of pee,
A chest X-ray and a doctor we did see.
Nothing glaring was found, and no more tests to do
So we left Saturday morning at a quarter to two.

Each day I feel a bit better as time goes by
With annoying things happening and I don't know why.
Like my left eye has randomly started to stick
Closed when I try to open it, a weird little trick.

I brushed my arm against the counter and felt
Pain so I looked and found a new welt.

Oh yea! It's phlebitis! And I don't know how
I even got it or what to expect now.

And this cough! Seriously, what's the deal?
Going on seven weeks now, and I feel
That it would be a hoot if next they found
That it is really pertussis that's going around!

Another caveat specific to me
Is odd with a capital O you see,
My EYEBROWS, both of them, are itchy and red,
At least the hair follicles are alive and not dead!

One third of my lash on my right has departed,
And no sign of any new hair growth has started.
Although they have thinned I still do have
A thin set of eyelashes; for that I am glad.

The list of the BS is part of the deal
Cancer treatment annoyances are definitely real.
But they not unbearable, and life is still good,
Life goes on, as I knew that it would.

The good news and yes, there is still some,
Is that my chemo treatments are now halfway done!
I start new drugs Thursday for the remaining four
Treatments will only be eight short weeks more.

I've been told that with Taxol I'll have an easier time
That the bone pain will be more in my hips and my thighs,
The infusion takes longer but they will start slow
To be sure I don't react badly or start to glow.

I can't believe it's December, this time is a blur
I'm already enjoying the season for sure.
At night when I sit beneath the Christmas tree lights,
I can be sure that I'm putting up a good fight.

Onward and upward, even with all the weird stuff
With all of my gifts I have more than enough.
My family's good health equals riches galore
For that I can't be happier and need nothing more!

CHAPTER FIFTEEN

New Drugs and New Information

Saturday, December 10, 2011

AFTER MY FOURTH round of chemo, I ended up in the Emergency Department. I was hurting from bone pain right after my Neulasta shot, and I felt awful, with hot flashes, a fever, and fatigue. Brian and I were shuffled quickly to a private room due to the chance of me being neutropenic (which meant I had a low white blood cell count, leaving me susceptible to infection) – and they didn't want me to be exposed to whatever germs were floating around in the waiting area. Two sets of blood cultures and labs were ordered, along with a chest X-ray and urinalysis.

The male nurse assigned to me had a difficult time when he tried to access my port to get my blood for labs. He was clearly nervous as he hummed and whistled and fumbled with equipment, and he tried accessing the port none too gently. Because I had this quirky thing where I could taste and smell the saline when the nurses flushed my IV or port, after he tried to flush, not one, not two, but *three* different times, I had to tell him that I could not taste the saline and therefore didn't believe he was in the port. Not to mention that with every flush that wasn't going into my port, the saline was going into my chest tissue, which stung.

The doctor on call that night finally made the executive decision to abort the standard "two blood cultures from separate sights" protocol. They had gotten one full sample from my arm, and that would prove to be enough for what they needed to do. My poor port was only four days old, and I was still sore from having it put in. After this experience, I wondered whether the port was difficult to access because of the nurse's bad luck or incompetence or because something was wrong with it. *Had something been dislodged? Would this lead to problems at my next round of chemo?*

Brain and I tried to find comfortable sleeping positions in the hard metal chairs as we waited for the results from my urine and blood cultures and chest X-ray. Finally at nearly 2:00 am, I was cleared to go. The final diagnosis was "Fever of unknown etiology." There was no clear finding as to what caused it, and naturally, my fever had magically gone down. They saw no medical reason to keep me there. We drove home exhausted, yet relieved.

A week and a half later, I realized that the difficult blood draw in the ED had planted a seed of uncertainty that compounded my anxiety level, because I was already anxious about starting my first dose of Taxol. (The first four rounds had been Adriamycin and Cytoxin, and the remaining four rounds would be a new drug called Taxol.) As I went in for the pre-chemo blood work, I really hoped that the port issues I'd had weren't a sign that the port was not patent. Thankfully, my pre-chemo blood draw was a piece of cake! The nurse was gentle and glided through the process with little to no effort at all. I had my interview with the oncology nurse next. She went through the nursing assessment, took notes, provided me with my lab results, and made sure all of my information and problem lists were up to date.

That day, a nurse practitioner was scheduled to see me because my regular oncologist was away on vacation.

The ARNP had been given the lowdown by the oncology nurse about my most recent concerns. She seemed warm and welcoming and easy to talk to. We started with my primary concern, which was this persistent cold that I had . . . runny nose, watery eyes, post-nasal drip, and a relentless cough triggered by talking, laughing, or any other little throat tickle. She matter-of-factly said (and *please*, take note of this in case you ever know someone going through this who thinks he or she can't shake a cold), "a side effect of chemo is cold-like symptoms, including post-nasal drip, that can result in a cough and a constant runny nose." I looked at Brian and shook my head. *Is she kidding me right now? How it is possible that I could be on round five of chemo and JUST find this out? Every week I mentioned this cold, this cough, this runny nose . . . . I was convinced I had whooping cough, for crying out loud! And all along, it was simply a side effect of chemo?* I thought of a set of sticky notes I saw at a store when I waited in the checkout line: "It burns 230 calories to bang your head on a wall for 15 minutes." *How long had I been banging my head against this wall?*

She suggested Claritin-D. *How could it be that simple?*

So, let's talk about Claritin-D for a second. The first weekend after chemo, when I experienced my first round of bone pain and fatigue, I went online to get an idea of how long the pain might last. What I found on a few websites were people writing on blogs saying, "I was told to take Claritin-D, and it significantly helped my bone pain." I saw it time and time again. Yet I couldn't figure out how the pharmacology worked – *why would an antihistamine and decongestant help with bone pain?* I called the on-call oncology nurse around the first week of treatment with a list of questions and concerns about mouth sores, body aches, hot flashes, because everything, at that point, was new to me. But I had also asked her back then about Claritin-D helping with bone pain, and she had never heard of it helping. I asked my local pharmacist, and he looked at me as if I'd been dipping hard into the narcotics.

So, when the nurse practitioner mentioned Claritin-D for my cold symptoms, the correlation popped back into my head, and I told her about what I had read. She confirmed that there was something to it (and I wasn't crazy!). As a matter of fact, a nurse practitioner used Claritin-D for bone pain in a study at Dartmouth-Hitchcock – and she was having great results! So, now I could take the Claritin-D for my cold symptoms AND see if it helped with the bone pain. I could kill two birds with one stone! What did I have to lose?

I hadn't really mentioned the issue of my eyelids sticking together, because I figured it was as unique to me as getting my period every other week. (Sigh.) Yes, 'tis true . . . my ovaries officially developed some form of dementia (self-diagnosed), and flip-flopped between menstruating and menopause. Every. Other. Fricken. Week. Coincidentally, as the ARNP continued talking about the cold-like symptoms, she made a natural transition to how people think cancer patients are crying because we have such leaky, gunky, or sticky eyes. I stopped her. "HEY! I HAVE THAT!" I'd wake up in the morning and try to open my eyes, and one would open, but the other wouldn't. (Brian started calling me Blinky.) She said it was because I didn't have a full set of eyelashes! Those little natural protectors of my eyes were thinning to almost non-existent (I could probably count the number of lashes that were left), and therefore could not do their job of keeping foreign particles out of my eyes. Hence, the tear ducts worked overtime to flush out foreign particles, leading my eyes to water and feel so gunky. I was SO glad I had a chance to talk with her! All of the little whiney things that had been accumulating were finally answered and justified! It was interesting to see how a different practitioner could shed light on so many different things.

After our appointment was through and all my questions were answered, Brian and I were escorted to Bay 3, where I'd spend the rest of the day. I would get three pre-meds, then the new chemo: Taxol. The three pre-meds were to help prevent an allergic reaction to the Taxol, which I was told was more common with this drug than the other two I had. They would start it off slowly, and I needed to watch for "anything out of the ordinary." This would have been much easier had I not gotten 50 mg of IV Benadryl. I've taken Benadryl by mouth before, and it did make me sleepy. But 50 mg right into my veins? Holy drunk and disorderly! I could barely keep my eyes open or speak after that went in. As my nurse was hanging my last pre-med, I looked at her and said, "Ifffeel like I'm drunk, Imso tired . . . ." I was aware of the Taxol going in but had by then reclined and gotten cozy with my heated blanket and pillow.

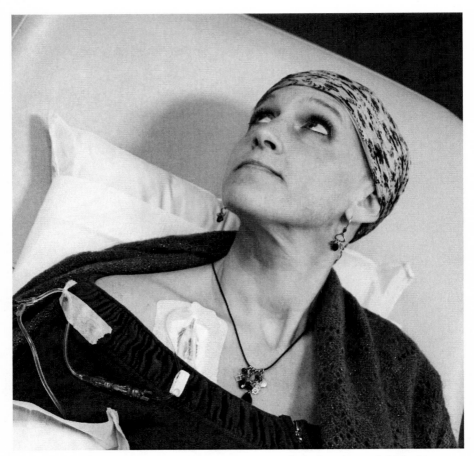

Chemotherapy infusion through my new port right before the meds kicked in

I was supposed to receive 200 cc of Taxol per hour, but they started it at 100 cc to see how I tolerated it. I guess sleeping – not moving yet still breathing – equated to "tolerating it well." So, they bumped me up to the normal administration rate for the remainder of the infusion. I was able to eat lunch and then was a barrel of laughs for Brian as he sat by me and I snoozed. I had started the day at 8:45 am with labs, and my infusion finished at 3:45 that afternoon. It was a long day.

Friday morning, I had a work meeting for the Physicians Association, followed by a few hours at the Coumadin Clinic, so I thought I'd give false eyelashes a whirl to help me feel a little more "put together." I had attempted them once before – EARLY in the morning, and they ended up stuck halfway up my left eyelid, so I aborted the mission then. But I decided to try them one more time.

Now, I didn't know the first thing about purchasing eyelashes. I was clearly no eyelash connoisseur. My thought process and methodology of picking them out went something like this: "Excuse me, where is your eyelash aisle? Aisle 5? Thank you." Find Aisle 5, where at least a half-dozen types of lashes sit on the rack – some short, some long, a full set, top and bottom, just bottom, an assembly of a dozen eyelash hair plugs (to be put on individually . . . like I'd have time for THAT!), extra full, then useless numbers of 103,105, 112 . . . whatever that means. I selected what looked like a top set of normal eyelashes compared to the others.

That Friday morning, I wrestled with them for a bit but got them on fairly straight, and they felt pretty good. They looked much thicker than my natural lashes did with mascara, but I figured that at the very least, they would detract from the no-hair and square-boob look I had going on. I surprised myself each time I looked in a mirror, thinking maybe I had chosen the Vegas Showgirl lashes by accident. All in all, it was a successful application.

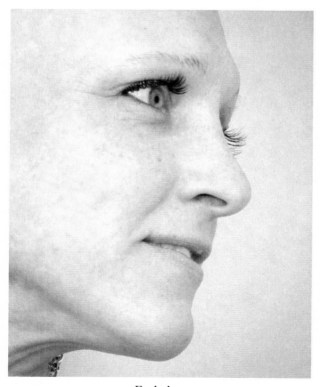

Eyelashes

However, by the time I headed home at 5 pm, about one-quarter inch of the outer corner of my right lashes were loose and stuck out to the side. I felt it with every blink. I don't think it was terribly noticeable to those around me, but to me, it looked as obvious as Tim Conway's toupee when he played Mr. Tudball on *The Carol Burnett Show*. Next time, I'd have to remember to bring additional adhesive or plan a shorter day.

Brian and I did a short photo shoot one Saturday. As usual, twenty-four hours after my Neulasta shot, I was in pain, fatigued, and on autopilot as I tried to cruise through the cumulative effects of chemo. This series of pictures captured me in a way I'd never experienced. I started off wearing my headscarf, then took that off and went to bald, then went even further by shedding my jewelry. For a series, I was bald, with no makeup, few eyelashes, no jewelry, and in a gray tee shirt. I'd never felt so exposed, yet I saw that the pictures captured the true essence of how it feels to go through this treatment when everything is stripped away – the pain, vulnerability, fear, exhaustion, and, regardless of the boundless support around me, the loneliness. That day's shoot was raw and real. I had asked Brian to take photos of as much of the positive as he could . . . after all, I'd been trying to keep things that way. The truth is, it WASN'T always positive, and I was entitled to feel overwhelmed at times. No one's life is without pain or challenges. This series of pictures reflected that feeling.

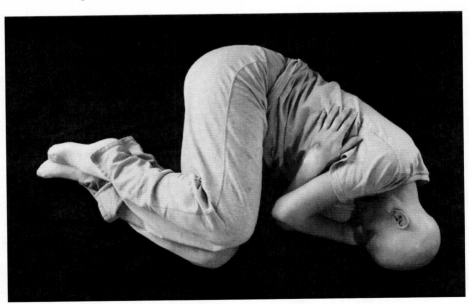

A painful down day

I kept taking the Claritin-D, and I think it helped to minimize the bone discomfort some, but not as much as I had hoped. The Taxol was supposed to contribute to a different type of joint/bone pain, so maybe taking it helped, and I just didn't realize the extent of it. Regardless, I laid low, taking pain meds as needed. I embraced my recovery time and waited for a new day to tackle.

CHAPTER SIXTEEN

Intimacy

Wednesday, December 28, 2011

CHEMOTHERAPY WAS NOW more than half over. It was in my system, it was wearing me down, and it was making me vulnerable in ways I discovered each day. It exhibited its effects in endless ways, the majority of which I was totally prepared for. Well, maybe I wasn't prepared for *exactly* what it would be like, but the nursing staff kept me well educated. I knew about the physical side effects – mouth sores, the possibility of joint aches, metallic taste, hair loss, fatigue – as well as the emotional side effects of feeling out of control, overwhelmed, and incapable to sort through it all when emotions mounted up. Plenty of literature was available to me on these problems, and the staff was always available to help provide suggestions or a compassionate, reassuring, listening ear. They heard similar versions of such frustrations and challenges on a regular basis, so their responses became second nature.

But I found other less common treatment-related issues that were essentially *breezed over* at my initial visit.

As I tried to keep on top of an abundance of new information, I really didn't think to question what *wasn't* covered in detail because, well, I couldn't anticipate EVERY possible thing that could happen. At every visit, I listened, took mental notes of what I might encounter, and filed it away.

Questions did arise as I heard about the possibilities of side effects. "How soon will my hair fall out?" or "What can I do about the metallic taste in my mouth?" Those questions are common and heard often and have pretty patented straightforward answers.

But I ran into some less common, more personal side effects. Ones that are not really discussed unless the patient brings them up, because they're uncomfortable, personal, or intimate. Ones that feel taboo.

The side effects I am referring to relate to sex and intimacy. There. I said it.

OK, let's just get this out there and on the table. I was a forty-three-year-old monogamous woman and a sexual being during my cancer treatment. I enjoyed, and still enjoy, everything about sex – from the connection it yields to how it makes me feel desirable to the snuggling afterwards. And, of course, both parties lying breathless and satisfied afterwards is the best part. Is this really that shocking? Can anyone really blame me? (This is where you shake your head "no" . . . come on; I'm going out on a limb here to share.) This is not a crazy, incomprehensible concept. It is part of who I am and nothing to be ashamed of. It is healthy and normal. So, why would it be so difficult to bring it up for discussion?

I think what it comes down to is that, for many reasons, sex and intimacy go to the bottom of the priority list when undergoing treatment. People are quite literally fighting for their lives. Some simply don't have the energy or desire to want anything but to feel better. And some may have partners who are too scared to broach the subject, let alone initiate anything. I believe that when you get down to brass tacks, if you are filled with toxins, controlling vomiting clearly trumps achieving an orgasm. Mustering the energy to initiate sex when you can barely make it to the bathroom to pee has as much likelihood as splitting the atom at the kitchen table. So, I reiterate, this subject lived somewhere at the bottom of the priority list. But it was still ON my list.

I realized that I had never really heard about cancer patients struggling with sexual concerns. So, I felt a little guilty, and it was weird that sex and intimacy was even **on** my radar. My friends and family watched me from a distance as I lost my hair, lived in the ebb and flow of the two-week increments between rounds of chemotherapy, and became more and more fatigued. They generously responded by offering their services to help me clean, mow my lawn, or make and deliver meals to the house. So would it all feel like a sham if they knew I was having sex on the days that I felt better? After all, if I had the energy for sex, shouldn't I have the energy to make dinner, too? Or at least prioritize which was more important?

In reality, I doubt that the thought really crossed anyone's mind but mine. The people who dropped off meals were not thinking that I waited by the door, looking tired and sick in my chemo cap and pink fuzzy robe and slippers, only to grab the food from them, toss it into the kitchen, and bolt upstairs, where I would drop my robe and reveal a negligee, garter, and feather boa before I hopped into the sack. (Truth be told, that doesn't even happen when I'm healthy.) But if they knew I was prioritizing my time to be intimate over cleaning or mowing or cooking dinner, would they feel I was taking advantage of them? It felt like a dirty little secret that I was hiding, which made me hesitant to bring it up.

My own issues aside, I think there's a juxtaposition that prohibits the discussion of sex and intimacy and the many challenges involved when going through treatment. It feels weird to waltz into an appointment with your oncologist and say, "You know what? I had a few hours the other day where I felt desirable and wanted intimacy, but I uncovered a number of issues and I'd like to discuss them." That is clearly not the norm. The medical staff is likely more concerned with the regular issues like, "How is your appetite? How is your pain? Are you moving your bowels all right? How are you sleeping?" When engulfed in such questions, there is no way to segue comfortably into what feels like an unworthy complaint of a new, irritating onset of vaginal dryness from the chemo-induced menopause. But when IS the right time?

I tried figuring it out on my own before bringing it up at an appointment. I often ask questions deeper than the average Jo, because I tend to delve into the etiology of different physical problems. I had been given a comprehensive cancer book for those with a medical background. It is detailed and informative, and on other occasions, it proved to be quite helpful. I scanned through it one day to see if it addressed any of my more specific intimacy issues. Boy Howdy, did it ever! Yikes! It outlined not only issues leading to trouble with intimacy, but also the staggering statistics about the inability to achieve an orgasm before, during, and after chemotherapy. The statistics were abysmal. I was almost one-hundred-percent certain that of the list of possible treatment side effects, "decreased ability to climax" had not been directly mentioned to me. I think I would have remembered that one.

It was likely lumped into the "vague-and-inexplicit-sexual-side-effects-to-be-explored-at-a-later-time-IF-the-need-arises" category. Although I was shocked at the data, I felt validated. *It wasn't just me! This was a real thing and likely just another side effect!* Now, I could identify that it was a real issue. And now, I needed some answers on how to fix it, because the book provided the depressing chart but no suggestions.

As I've mentioned, there are many very good reasons why discussing sex and intimacy takes a back seat. It's personal, it's intimate, and the fear of being judged by what you do behind closed doors makes a person feel very vulnerable. But it is still important. As a nursing student, I remember the lectures where we first learned the importance of acknowledging that, regardless of age, every person is a sexual being. My initial reaction was, *Good Lord, really? Old people getting their groove on? Thanks for* that *visual. What does this have to do with nursing?* The answer is, it has *a lot* to do with nursing. When a person is going through an illness, the burning question is, "How will this affect my life? What will I have to change? What will be different?" Nurses and medical professionals are caring for the whole person and that person's subsequent quality of life. They need to be prepared to answer these questions without judgment. Our job is to help people attain the best quality of life they can. We do that by allowing patients to discuss and ask questions about *anything*. We may not have an immediate answer, but we can find some bit of information to help allay their concerns. Although I don't know specific statistics, I tend to believe that if I have sex questions, there are probably a lot more people out there who also have questions but don't know the right time or place to ask them.

Although it generally goes without saying that sex changes during cancer treatment, I will tell you the specifics of what I found to be true for me.

First, and most obviously, my body changed physically. I had expanders for breasts that both looked and felt awkward. They were hard, they didn't move, and I had no feeling in them, except for an underlying residual surgical pain. I didn't feel soft and curvy; I felt hard and lumpy. Sometimes I'd take a corner too fast (especially when I was on meds that affected my balance), the expanders would hit the wall, and literally, the only thing I felt was the cessation of forward momentum. For cases like that, having no feeling was an advantage. But when it came to what my square boobs brought to the table for intimate moments, not so much. They might as well have had yellow-and-black police tape draped across them that read, "Caution: Crime Scene. Do Not Enter. Detour, Head South." When I made the decision to have both breasts removed, I knew that losing feeling in my nipples would be a loss. However, I hadn't really put much thought into how creative and open-minded I would need to be to fill that void. Without sensation in my breasts, it felt as I'd gone from broadband to dial-up. What was once seamless, easy, and instantaneous was now unfamiliar, difficult, and painfully slow, making me wonder if I'd ever get to an end point. It could be done, but I had to be patient because it took much longer to reach my goal.

Next, there was the fact that I was bald. Feeling sexy with a glaring, shiny head was a challenge for me. Not to mention that "batting my eyelash" in a coy fashion clearly did not have the same seductive effect as batting a full set. The upside was that I didn't have to spend any time shaving; my legs, armpits, and all related "grooming areas" were taken care of naturally by the chemo.

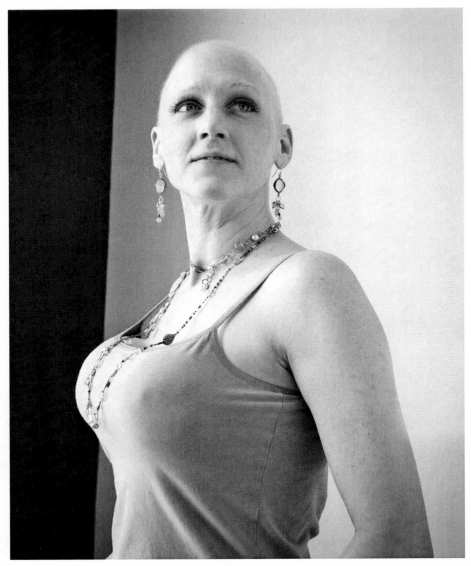

Bald with expanders

Scars adorned my body – on my sides from the drains, on my breasts from the surgery, on my chest where an acorn-sized lump sat from the port.

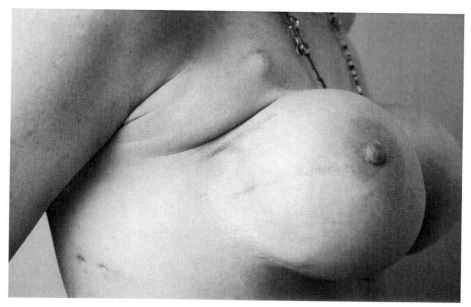

What I saw every day . . .

My skin pallor was also off somehow. Although it *was* winter in New England, and turning pasty white is part of the normal cycle for us Yankees, chemotherapy left me with a sickly pallor. The familiar body I once had was replaced with a foreign one. All in all, there were moments where I couldn't help but feel I looked like a train wreck with all of these unwelcome alterations.

The icing on the cake was that with the cumulative effects of chemotherapy, I had a lower threshold of acceptance and patience. It was comparable to what happens when an overtired toddler hears "no" and falls apart to the extent that the reaction is grossly disproportional to the precipitating event. The same went for me. The toxins that fought off cancer cells in my body took a lot out of me. I was tired, whether I wanted to admit it or not. So, what may not seem like a big deal to anyone else felt monumental to me. I had to stay mindful that I was vulnerable because of a combination of fatigue, toxins, and changing hormones. I tried to remember that things were probably not as bad as they sometimes felt.

But wait! There's more! Once I addressed the hurdles of *feeling* attractive, there were the physical issues of what menopause left behind in its wake. Menopause is not just surges of hot flashes. It's a woman's body telling her it's time to retire from child bearing. The eggs released from her ovaries no longer slide down the slippery fallopian tubes at full speed, like a child on a water slide heading for the pool at the bottom. Instead, they shuffle down in orthopedic shoes, with little egg walkers, carefully hobbling down one step at a time. And simultaneously, the well of lubrication proceeds to dry up. Reinforcements need to be called in.

Normally, Mother Nature allows this natural process to take its time gradually, over a span of years. In the case of chemo-induced menopause, the body is jolted into this transition, and BAM! It's done. Before you can even say, "Astroglide," rude and unwelcome changes have already taken place. It is quick, it is jarring, and it is intense. What it's NOT is forgiving. And it is yet another hurdle to jump over when trying to feel attractive, sexy, or, at the very least, familiar.

So, I asked myself, *now that I have found this accumulation of issues, how do I address them?* I needed to find out which issues had alternative solutions and which ones I'd have to live with. It was time for another sit down heart-to-heart with my oncologist.

Thankfully, my oncologist totally got it. She wasn't afraid to address anything. I asked her about everything I could think of, and she made me feel at ease and comfortable. In fact, when I brought up the intimacy and sexual issues I was having, part of me secretly thought that maybe there was a part of her thinking, "You GO, girl! Keep it real!" because she was so supportive and understanding.

As a practice, my oncologist checked in and talked with me before the actual infusion at every chemo visit. She wanted to ensure that all was well before proceeding. The morning of my sixth treatment, I was told that she was seeing one patient before me and that she would come over to see me after that. The nurses started infusing the pre-meds as I waited. The first one was an IV steroid called Decadron, and the other was IV Benadryl, given over a half-hour or so.

As the Benadryl infused, I quickly became utterly EXHAUSTED. I danced in and out of sleep. I was aware of noises around me (which always yield weird dreams), and therefore could respond briefly to general questions asked by the nursing staff. It felt as if I were drunker than drunk. I slurred my words even though I attempted, with all my might, to articulate. My eyes felt weighted down with lead. If I was asked a question that required an answer of more than five words, no matter how I tried to maintain eye contact, my weighted lids would steadily close, and I would drift off to sleep within seconds.

Unfortunately, this was when my oncologist came by to talk to me.

When she asked me how things were going, it took all of my memory power to remember that I wanted to address the intimacy issues. I propped my eyelids open with my fingers, and I mentioned that I was having some struggles with lubrication and was frustrated with trying to be intimate. She didn't bat an eye. She said there were things I could try that might help, but they didn't come without caution. I heard her talking and tried to stay engaged in the conversation, but she sounded like the teacher in Charlie Brown specials. She said she would write me a script and to call her if I developed any questions. She left the script at my side.

After discharge that day, I had the script in hand and headed to the pharmacy to have it filled. But, when I got home, I realized that I didn't remember much about my conversation with her. I read the warnings and contraindications on the accompanying pharmacy paperwork and became mildly alarmed. When I saw that the medication was contraindicated for women with breast cancer, I could vaguely recall that she had addressed this, but since I didn't remember the specifics of what she'd said, I decided to call her.

She immediately took my call, and we reviewed our previous conversation. The medication was Estring, a ring that is inserted vaginally and gives off low, local doses of estrogen to help stimulate natural lubrication. It's often prescribed for post-menopausal women. Encouraging any form of estrogen with a patient whose cancer feeds off it is clearly risky. However, she reiterated that although there were very small doses of estrogen given off from this ring, it was localized and not systemic (meaning it would stay put in the vaginal area and would not spread around my whole body). This was one of those medications that did not have a lot of conclusive research studies. There was no data proving that women who used Estring experienced higher recurrence rates of cancer, nor any data that showed it didn't. She said it could be placed and left for three months, or I could put it in for a shorter time to see if it was effective and use it in shorter intervals.

So, there were the facts: my oncologist was comfortable recommending it, and there were no studies that said that it would definitely increase my chance for recurrence. If the normalcy of natural lubrication was important to me, then, it was a risk I could take. It was important to take quality-of-life issues seriously and worthwhile to address things that made me feel as normal as possible. She said they did track all patients who had been prescribed this medication, though, so I would be contacted if any significant findings would contraindicate using it after further studies.

I hung up the phone and was overwhelmed with information. It was probably the effects of the earlier chemo, but I felt torn, lost, and defeated. I had wanted options. She gave me one. Now I wanted a better option. Nothing was easy. I sat at the counter and cried. Why did every decision have to be so hard?

Brian and I talked it through. He was on the other side of the debate. He didn't see the sense in even taking the chance to put me more at risk for recurrence. I told him I didn't feel desirable. Not that sitting there with a runny nose, red swollen eyes, and a general depressive demeanor was helping my cause any. He told me that I *was* desirable . . . and beautiful. He said that when I was feeling a little better, we should do a photo shoot; he would prove to me how beautiful I was.

Sometimes, you have to think out of the box. Sometimes, you have to embrace something unfamiliar and slightly out of your comfort zone to get out of a funk. Sometimes, striving for "the same" becomes far too frustrating, and you have to go in the opposite direction and do something totally different.

For example, my wig choice. I cherished the time that I spent with Lisa when we picked out my wig. We tried to get a look that would make me feel like myself and make me comfortable. But every time I put it on, it was just different enough from my old haircut that it looked as if I were trying too hard.

So, I decided to go longer. Go bold. Go totally different. I knew that I didn't have the patience to grow my hair out, so if ever there was an opportunity for me to embrace long hair, it was now. What was the worst that could happen? People would laugh? So, I ended up getting one mid-length, brown-hair wig. This wig and a pair of false eyelashes and once again, I felt sassy, alive, and reborn!

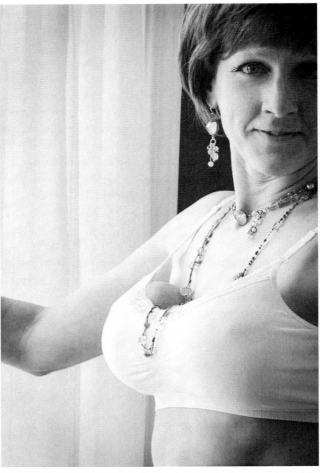

Wig, eyelashes and expanders . . . feeling a little more desirable

As for feeling beautiful, well, I needed to go in a different direction yet again and think out of the box. The Saturday morning following my sixth treatment, Brian had me pick out my favorite headscarf and put it on and await further instruction. As he disappeared, I put on eyelashes and a bit of makeup, a pair of heels. He was thinking outside of the box, all right. He returned with a box of Saran Wrap. *What on earth are we going to do with that?* "Trust me," he said.

He found the end of the Saran and proceeded to wrap me around and around and around, starting at my bust and working his way down to the middle of my thighs. Although the wrap might be see-through enough to identify food when storing leftovers, on my body it left a crinkly white texture with a little skin color peeking through. It comfortably covered enough so that "intimate" details were hidden, revealing nothing but a shimmery silhouette. He grabbed his camera and started taking pictures. It was a PG-13 photo shoot that concentrated solely on making me feel sexy and desirable, and initially thought it would be for our eyes only. Completely bald, I was finally able to let my hair down. With my flaws covered, I felt like a star, like a model; I felt more beautiful than I had in ages.

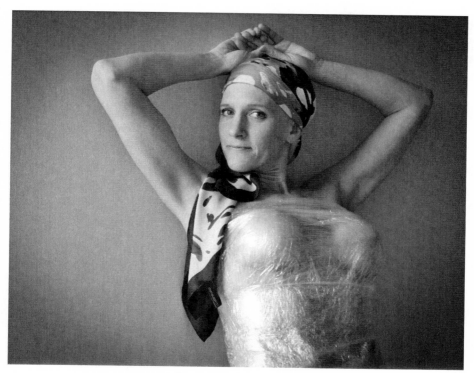

Saran wrap photo shoot

We reviewed the pictures. Brian had perfectly captured the joy I'd been feeling, and even I could see how happy I was, and how, for that brief period of time, I wasn't a cancer patient. I was America's next top model. I'd spent so much time getting lost in treatment that I lost sight of how to make my inner beauty shine. Up until then, I was desperately trying to find the old me, not realizing that this "new" me was just the old me with a lot of stuff piled on top. It was buried just under the surface of anticipation of what I would encounter next on this journey and how I would handle it.

As well as I thought I was handling things, I still had "Ah-ha!" moments that jarred me out of my cancer fog. That photo shoot was one of those moments. It boosted my self-esteem and reminded me that I *was* desirable. The intimacy issues would only resolve if I relaxed and tried not to add the stress of trying to fix it at a time when I wasn't at one hundred percent.

Intimacy was yet another area where I had to give myself a break. It couldn't be the same at that point, just like my body couldn't be the same; another reality I had to accept. Even though accepting things as temporary was a recurring theme, it always felt like an epiphany when I re-realized it. I would give myself a break. And be sure to keep Saran Wrap on my shopping list.

CHAPTER SEVENTEEN

I've Lost That New Cancer Smell

Monday, January 2, 2012

A NEW CAR is exciting. Who doesn't love sliding into one, the excitement of getting to know the way it handles, adjusting the controls and understanding the new instrument panel, cranking up the stereo (even the music sounds better!) and, oh yeah, that incredible new car smell! You swear this car will be different; it will stay new, and it will be taken care of properly. You establish the "new car rules": No food, (especially crackers and crumbly stuff), no smoking, no leaving your stuff in the back seat, and no dirt on your shoes before you get in (you have to keep the floor mats clean, after all). When it's new, you even notice when a little white gum wrapper is left behind, because it taints the order of the flawless interior. You remain vigilant, because you're reminded of the importance of keeping everything clean, neat, and nice every time you slide in and smell that new car smell.

Inevitably, you rush to work one morning, and coffee splashes out of the mouth hole of the seemingly spill-proof mug – all down the front of the console – and you scramble for some form of napkin (of course, you have sworn off hoarding extra napkins in this car to avoid the clutter). With one hand, you do your best, but you don't have the time to clean it up properly. You are asked at the last minute to pick up your son's best friend from baseball, and the two of them hop into the back seat – all their gear scattered everywhere – and the dirt from their cleats finds a comfortable resting place deep in the rug floor mats. You park next to an SUV at the store and come out to find a ding in the driver side door. It's not enough to fix, just enough to totally irk you every time you look at it. A random light comes on to notify you that there is a malfunction somewhere, and although the car is under warranty, you now have to budget your time around dropping it off to have it fixed.

As you fill it with gas one day, you glance in the back seat and spot contraband: baggies with crumbs, a Gatorade bottle on the floor with two swallows of purple liquid left in it, your daughter's sneakers, the baseball hat your son couldn't find, and his friend's jacket that was randomly left behind. And gum wrappers everywhere.

None of these things are catastrophic or make you love it any less. "Life" has happened to your car. The new car smell has worn off. Now, you find yourself simply doing your best to maintain it the best you can as you accept the dings, the clutter, and the coffee drip on the console.

Now, forget the new car. Eyes here. I discovered that my new cancer smell had worn off.

In the beginning, I was surrounded by an overwhelming plethora of healthcare team members. It felt as if they were everywhere I turned. They said they could cure the cancer; there was a plan; I would be fine; it would be a long haul, but on the other side, all would be well. I was the star of the show! I had surgical oncologists, genetic counselors, medical oncologists (residents and attending), nurses doing lymphedema studies, radiation oncologists, my primary care doctor, my general surgeon, my gyn doctor, and all of the people doing tests, drawing blood and checking me in and out of facilities, paying attention to me. I had that new cancer smell. I felt like the refried beans wrapped in the middle of a cancer survivor burrito, the caterpillar nestled in the cocoon of hope. I was the middle fish in a school of support and strategy. I was the star of the new reality show, *Tracy vs. Cancer*. My medical peeps were everywhere. I felt so protected.

At the beginning of this discovery phase, as I tried to process all that was happening, naturally, word got out to the masses. It started with family and close friends, then friends of the kids, and then came the trickle-down effect. Support galore. Meals overflowing the fridge and freezer, a constant string of phone calls, unvarying offers to help, and the mail . . . oh, the mail . . . when fun mail outweighs the bills, and even magazines, you know you are supported.

When managing cancer treatment is new, there are obvious tasks like visits, meals, and schedules to manage. Those tasks are the ones that can be challenging but don't have catastrophic effects if not tended to or addressed. An example: early on, I realized that I had to eat but didn't have much of an appetite the weekend after chemo due to a metallic taste, mouth sores, and a simple lack of desire. Friends and family by nature wanted to help, so I requested light meals for those few days. This worked for a few rounds until I realized that as much as the soup, salad, and quiches I requested were wonderful, it was just as easy to grab a bowl of cereal or a piece of toast. I didn't imagine that it would feel quite as rewarding to deliver a box of Cinnamon Life and a quart of milk to my doorstep as it would be to make a nice healthy salad and homemade soup. But I guess that depended on who prepared the meal. You know who you are, and I love you.

Then there were the less-than-obvious things like physical symptoms and the side effects from the side effects to manage. Example: managing the increased pain from the combination of the Taxol and Neulasta shot. If I took a narcotic, it helped ease the pain, but it was constipating, so I also took a stool softener. I was started on Decadron, a steroid, to help ease the pain and perhaps lessen the number of narcotics I needed. It helped more than anything else did, but it too had its own set of side effects, like making me hungry and thirsty, which I hadn't noticed until I stepped on the scale and discovered the weight gain. And let's touch on the emotional liability? Four words. *Whoa and holy shit.* I was in tears every day. No, not from the weight gain, but unpredictably, pretty much from anything and everything else life had to offer – the degree of the earth's axis and the speed of its rotation, the temperature of the soup I had for lunch, trying to match a scarf with my outfit. But the kicker on top of that was the awesome case of insomnia that made me overtired *and* emotional. Perfect. So I took Xanax to help me sleep. Was it worth it? Yes, it totally was. Was it absolutely ree-freakin-diculous that I took pills to counteract the side effects of pills I took for my symptoms? Yes, but it was temporary, and kind of like a fun little "pill puzzle." (Eye roll.)

I was told that a healthy body is resilient. That it will bounce back from the craziness of chemo and all of its drug companions' side effects as all of the cancer cells are dying off, thinking, "Good Lord, what is happening here? We can't handle a host that is so unpredictable!"

But, there are a number of things that no one really tells you about the cancer journey, and therefore, it took me longer to understand and figure some of them out. Setting the physical elements aside, I identified a few key predictable unpredictable consistencies. (Yes, I meant to say that.) These issues were chameleon-like – they constantly changed their color to blend into the next situation, just when I thought I understood them. It made asking for help virtually impossible, because I couldn't anticipate my need until it stared me in the face. That's where I was in my journey – figuring out what was happening physically and emotionally, then trying to deal with it. More specifically, I realized what the healthcare team doesn't prepare you for is the real meaning of "living through cancer treatment."

I know all the specifics can't be laid out, because everyone is different, and no one can anticipate how each individual will respond to treatment. But I identified and broke down three predictably unpredictable and frustrating situations that are underrated:

1. Understanding (my) Emotions and Feelings
2. Dealing with the Oncological Purgatory – Waiting (aka Healing time)
3. Embracing Body Image (Or, Trying to, at Least)

Understanding Emotions & Feelings

I was told to be prepared for being sick and tired of being sick and tired somewhere around two-thirds of the way through chemotherapy. I officially was. But I use that term loosely. Although I wasn't vomiting sick, bouncing back from my bad days, after a number of cycles, took a lot out of me. I am eternally grateful that in my chemo regimen, I actually felt pretty good seventy-five percent of the time.

I had to redefine "good," though. I told people I felt *mostly* back to normal. But it was a Cancer Normal, or, more positively speaking, a Transitional Normal, not a Tracy Normal. And I was not fully prepared for the emotional intensity and management of the Transitional Normal.

On my "bad" days, I pretty much wrote off the Friday night after chemo until the following Tuesday afternoon. I didn't plan anything big; I didn't operate heavy machinery, play with knives, sign important life-changing documents, or set goals other than to remember to take my pills, drink fluids, and eat. Work took a back seat, because those days were officially set aside for nothing more than healing. The bad days, thankfully, were short lived. They were not the end of the world, and although I didn't necessarily look *forward* to them, I didn't *dread* them, either. I *did* look forward to knowing that I got "one more down," and that would make it tolerable.

But, as I came back to life, I realized I'd essentially lost four days of getting anything worthwhile done. Although I told myself it was OK to take the time to heal, when I felt better, I also felt the need to make up for lost time.

I was only back to Transitional Normal, though. In a Tracy Normal day, I didn't have residual joint pain, swing between constipation and diarrhea, battle insomnia, experience neuropathy in my feet and hands, have sticky eyes, go through hot flashes, and, let's all say it together on the count of three . . . one, two, three . . . *sport square boobs*. (I know. I beat that one to death.) In a Tracy Normal day, it didn't take me more than an hour to get ready for work, nor would I yearn for a nap by 2 pm. (Well, OK, maybe I would love a nap normally, but I certainly wouldn't hit a wall by then.) No matter what, I put on my game face, made the best of what I could (and couldn't) do, kept an optimistic outlook, put a fancy bow on it, and Ta-Daaaaa! I reached Transitional Normal! It was certainly better than the bad days, but even when I was at one-hundred percent of my Traditional Normal, I was still only at eighty percent of my Tracy Normal. I was . . . trying . . . but . . . Just. Couldn't. Get. There.

My oncologist told me that when I hit my final chemo treatment, it might bring mixed feelings. Going through an established routine every other week, seeing the familiar faces at the cancer center, knowing there was an active plan to rid me of evil rogue cancer cells that might try to find a home, would suddenly end. Then, there would be no active treatment. I'd swim in that vast ocean I mentioned earlier, but the current would whisk me away from my school of support and strategy, and I'd find myself swimming alone. I'd be on stage, and the spot light would go off, and I'd hear someone's solitary voice echo, "That's a wrap." (Single person applauding . . . clap . . . clap . . . clap.) *But wait, I haven't even made it through the second act!* Although I would start radiation therapy in another four-to-six weeks, nothing really prepared me for how to deal with the wait, the down time, the "you-look-good-and-aren't-doing-anything-to-actively-FIGHT-cancer-so-you-must-be-back-to-normal" phase, where expectations increased, yet I was still in Transitional Normal. *Helloooo? Anyone seen my cancer survival burrito? And why are there so many gum wrappers around me?*

Enough time had passed so that treatments and healing time were now part of the routine, and the shock and awe of a new cancer diagnosis had worn off. Because nothing catastrophic happened (thank God) – I didn't have any complications or die – it seemed I was doing just fine. Sometimes, putting a smile on your face and trying to be brave backfires. Although things could have been much worse, in many ways, I was pretty far from "fine." I TOTALLY lost my new cancer smell. Damn.

I knew that I had to accept what life was offering me. Life was happening – not how I pictured it, like keeping a car all shiny and new – but I saw the dents and felt the reality and fatigue of healing and therefore, I had to lower my expectations a bit. There. I said it. This initially felt like defeat, but contrary to popular belief, I knew I had put a lot of pressure on myself to keep up with everything, and I tried to do so with a smile on my face. I *had* given myself permission to heal, but I did need to be reminded on occasion that it was OK if I didn't sweat the small stuff. All right . . . OK . . . I still needed to be reminded *often*. But I was a work in progress.

Dealing with the Oncological Purgatory – Waiting (aka Healing Time)

The time between treatments feels like an Oncological Purgatory. You're not actively in treatment, but you need time to heal or recover before you can do anything more. This purgatory feels closer to hell than heaven . . . I'm just sayin'. Frieda and I agreed that "waiting" time is like this: Life *doesn't actually* stop, although it sort of *feels as if* it does. The show must go on. I had to embrace the fact that even though my hair might be growing back, which was good, it wasn't *really* back.

It would still be a while before I didn't LOOK and feel like a cancer patient. So I penciled in eyebrows, decided if I should coat the few lashes I had with mascara or don the fake ones, and tried to find clothes that fit my altered body to make me feel confident. I headed to work and interacted with people at my job who had no idea what I'd just been through or how I was mentally struggling as I had to wait, surrounded by gum wrappers, pretending that all was well.

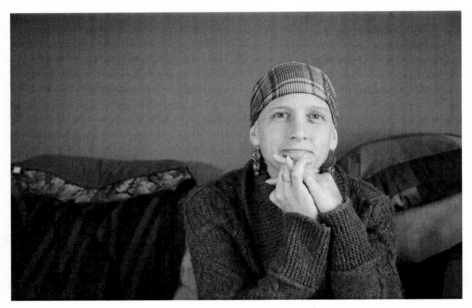

pretending everything is normal

It felt as if I'd witnessed a massive 747 crash on the side of the road on my way to work. I could see the plane engulfed in flame, metal pieces everywhere, people groaning and crying as they limped out of the carnage. It was unbelievable, but there was nothing I could do as I drove by – it was done and over, and I could only be horrified by the sight of it all, unable to shake the memory of what I witnessed. So, when I got to work and I talked on the phone or emailed insurance companies and doctors' offices, it was difficult to focus, because all I wanted to do was interrupt a conversation and say, "Did you hear about that horrific plane crash on the side of the road?"

I know. It seems unprofessional to bring up the crash, because it is obviously not relevant to work . . . and yeah, OK, there is that small detail that it didn't *really* happen. But it felt *so real* to me. It made me feel as if I were living in an alternate world, because no one but me had any knowledge about it. *How could that be? It was HUGE . . . shouldn't it be all over the news? How could I concentrate on everything I needed to do when I was thinking about those injured people? Those flames . . . the fact that it happened on my way to work . . . .*

It stuck in my head. It was stuck there. I knew it was there, but others didn't. And no matter how I might try to describe it to someone who hadn't seen it too, they'd never be able to understand fully what it was like.

My cancer treatment held the same weight as that non-existent plane crash. To get through this, I realized that I needed to find other people who saw or experienced the crash, too. For me, it helped to talk about it and not feel so alone, so crazy. Those people were other survivors – other men and women who had been through their own crashes and who understood firsthand. Yes, I reached out to find out about the local breast cancer support group and discovered co-workers who'd been to it. They were reassuring as they said to me, "I saw it too. It's scary. But, the worst is over. The people from the crash all walked away OK."

Part of recovery is acknowledging the support of those who have been there and have seen their own "crash." Those trained professionals and close friends will support and listen when you just need to say and hear in return, "Yeah, this part really sucks."

Embracing Body Image

At the beginning of all of this, when all of the doctors were actively sharing their ideas and treatment plans, I was embraced in hope and perhaps a false sense of security. I thought that providers would tenderly hand me off with kid gloves to one another like a fragile egg. The surgical oncologist would perform the mastectomy and gingerly pass me to the plastic surgeon, who would put in the expanders and follow and monitor me until my chemotherapy. Then the medical oncologist would tenderly take me and follow me through the chemo and pass me off to the radiation oncologist, who would complete the circle by gently passing me back to the plastic surgeon, when, finally, I'd be as ready as I could to go out on my own.

Survey says? Ehhhhhh! As it turns out, I was the walking oncological version of Mrs. Potato Head.

Picture the potato.

It started with my surgical oncologist, who took off my breasts, and I woke with eyes, ears, a mouth, and hands to start. Not arms and hands . . . just hands. With these four things, I could hear the plan, ask questions, and see what needed to be done. With no arms, I couldn't reach too far, but I could get the *basics* done. I was then tossed, hot potato style, from the surgical oncologist to the plastic surgeon. She put on little bumps for my breasts and then added feet. Again, not legs, just feet, and she said, "Don't do too much," as if I could do anything with feet directly attached to my body but no legs. With each "fill," I noticed the actual *placement* of each of my breasts. Huh. One was placed in the middle of my forehead and the other on my chest. There was nothing I could do but try to make them look normal.

The time between my surgery and when I met my oncologist, still weeks away from starting chemotherapy, I wasn't passed off to anyone. I was put away on a shelf in my own little world, left to figure out how to deal with the changes going on in my body. (Please refer back to the "waiting phase.") After a long, dark month on this shelf, I met my medical oncologist. She started me on chemo, which took my hair, eyelashes, and eyebrows. (Are you still picturing the potato?) But, she actually gave me one arm! Now, I could do more, but not quite everything I could before surgery.

After eight rounds of chemo (only two more doses to go!), this bald, strangely arranged Mrs. Potato Head was put back on the shelf to deal with the wait . . . again. Sure, I'd try on sunglasses and attempt to grow another arm and perhaps legs too, in order to try to do more until I was tossed into whatever changes radiation would bring. I might have been a tough, adapting potato on the outside, but I felt like a fragile egg on the inside.

It was time to figure out how the potato and the egg could merge to make something palatable. I had no choice but to accept this look and let my attitude be my guide. Everything was temporary. It would all be normal again. I just had to keep finding ways to polish my inner beauty until after my final surgery in the summer, when not only would my breasts be fixed, but I would officially (and FINALLY) be given arms to embrace a new, cancer-free life, and legs to keep moving forward.

Yes, I had lost my new cancer smell; I may not have had a plethora of medical and surgical teams gingerly passing me off at every new juncture, but I see now that was because I could take it. I AM a tough potato, WITH a delicate egg interior – one that had to set realistic goals, share the scary stuff, and rely on inner peace.

There's a reason the big-lipped smile was stuck on my Mrs. Potato Head. Because in the dark hours, when dealing with yet another "you've-got-to-be-kidding-me" moment, a big-lipped smile is what I had to fall back on.

CHAPTER EIGHTEEN

The Game Changer

Tuesday, January 17, 2012

AFTER I RETURNED from the Navy, I had a few months off and then resumed a part-time, evening position at a local hospital. It was my favorite shift, always my best time to shine, but hard on family life. So, when I was offered a full-time day job, no weekends, no holidays, with decent pay, I took it, not realizing that as a mother, I had signed up for two full-time jobs. (Ask any full-time working mother.) There were meals, homework, shopping, cleaning, transportation from one event to the next . . . and, dare I say, no time to exercise or have quality time to relax or have family fun. I remember trying to swing into the store (shopping) on the way home from soccer (transportation from event) to grab one last item in order to be able to whip together the easiest dinner I could think of (meal) that might have more nutritional value than the box it came in. The girls would do their out-loud nightly reading to me (homework) while I picked up (cleaning), and the only "exercise" I got was from running up and down the stairs getting kids ready for bed before I headed to bed myself at eleven pm (time to relax). I had accomplished everything I needed to do. But did it really count? Was I really doing anything well? Doing the bare minimum to keep things going isn't very satisfying. Yet if I concentrated on doing one thing well, everything else went to hell in a hand basket.

My life during cancer treatment felt a bit like that. I barely squeaked by trying to do my normal things; I accomplished the bare minimum but did nothing well. I felt defeated, as though I'd failed. Defeat tasted bitter; failure smelled pungent. And, alas, I was only halfway through and already feeling this way. That wasn't good, and I knew I needed a plan.

Alcoholics, smokers, and other addicts need to admit there's a problem before they can get on the road to recovery. I knew I felt overwhelmed, out of control, frustrated, tired, and vulnerable. I knew I needed an outlet; I needed to talk to people who understood this journey. So I picked up the phone and made two calls. One was to the social worker, Ann, at the cancer center. She gave me the date and time of the next breast cancer support group. The second was to my personal counselor.

As I walked in to the first support group meeting, I had two conflicting emotions: worry and hope. Worry: *Would I leave still feeling isolated? What if I cried? Would they judge me?* Hope: *We all have a common denominator; cancer has chosen us and changed our lives, so this must be a safe place to share.* The group consisted of seven of us: Ann, the social worker, who was the intuitive and thoughtful coordinator and leader of the meeting; one woman who was going through treatment similar to mine and who brought a friend for support; one woman who was more than a year out of treatment but still navigating through complications; two survivors who were a few years out; and me. We were each to introduce ourselves and tell a little about our story before we started "discussions."

As someone in the middle of treatment, with expanders still in place, I was in a spot where I still didn't know how I would feel or look after all of this was over and my final surgery was done. So, as the first woman introduced herself and said, "I had a lumpectomy with radiation treatment and no reconstruction," I found myself looking at her face . . . then instinctively at her breasts. *Whoops! Whoa! Oh my gosh, what did I just do? Avert your eyes! That was so rude! OK, collect yourself Tracy, don't do that again.* The next woman who talked had a lumpectomy, chemo, radiation, and reconstruction, and also had a lift and partial implants in her other breast as well. She did the 'ole right-shoulder-forward, left-shoulder forward move that brought attention to her chest as she described her reconstruction. So, I looked, again, this time just to be polite. I think.

At that point, I realized it was pretty normal to meet these women head-on with a smile and then check out their busts. Their breasts were just as individual as their faces, and it felt OK and safe to look, because (1) I knew they knew how it felt to be in my shoes, and perhaps years ago when they were going through it, they were curious too, (2) there was comfort in seeing a "survivor" come to a meeting to show, both with attitude and appearance, that things become normal again, to the point where no one could tell they'd ever undergone cancer treatment, and (3) I realized that I'd lost count of how many times I had to reveal my breasts to healthcare professionals, and although it was extremely personal to me, I was just another patient to them. Although I was always aware of a level of discomfort when a new provider needed to look at – or, worse yet, manipulate – my breasts, I built a wall of tolerance to it. I had to let go of feeling humiliated or embarrassed, because it wasn't sexual, it was methodical and necessary.

These women knew how that felt too, so what was one more person looking? My turn came to introduce myself. *Sit up straight, shoulders back, knockers out. Ten bucks says they will sneak a peek at mine, too. It is what it is.*

However, shocking as it may be, boob gazing was not the reason I went to the support group. Ann got the conversation started. I believe, based on a conversation I had had with her three weeks before, that she must've taken notes or remembered my concerns, or maybe it was pure coincidence. But the topics she brought up hit home – it was as if she opened up my heart and head, and all of my feelings spilled out onto the table. Things like, "How do you tell people that you just can't handle everything after they tell you that you look so good? As someone who rarely asks for help, how do you say that you just can't do whatever it is you've been asked to do? How do you lower your expectations of yourself without feeling as if you are failing?" *Yeah, how do you adjust your thinking to where it's OK to do the bare minimum and accept that for right now, that IS enough? And why the hell am I crying so much? How do I make it stop? Is it the steroids alone, or are these symptoms just worsened by them? Has anyone else noticed an emotional rollercoaster or 'roid rage while taking them? Seriously, why don't the steroids come with a warning on the label stressing the hazards of operating power tools under their influence?*

I need to take a little side trip here that has nothing to do with the support group, except that we discussed the effects of steroids on our emotions. My oncologist suggested that I try taking the steroid Dexamethasone to help ease my bone pain. I had nothing to lose, so I started taking them one Friday after chemo.

One weekend, I was double dipping, taking the steroids and narcotics for pain. This combination altered my decision-making abilities into thinking that *putting up window treatments* would be a good, and maybe even *fun*, idea. So, on day two of taking steroids, I tried it. Picture this: It's high noon. It's me, the window treatment, hardware, and a power drill. After coaxing a tight fitting, uncooperative mounting board into the inside molding of Abbie's bedroom window, I felt a rage start in my toes and work its way up my body. *Why wasn't this easier?* I started having off-the-charts-intense hot flashes and, as a result, began to disrobe. I peeled off my headscarf and whipped it across the room with the intense force of, well, a scarf being thrown across the room (very unsatisfying for unloading frustration). I then progressed to the outermost layers of clothes. One by one, sweatshirts, slippers, and socks were sent flying in all directions. I admonished and swore at my clothing for being so inconsiderately hot and for the inconvenience of making me sweat as though that were the very reason for their existence.

I returned to the installation. The weight in the bottom of the window treatment repeatedly clunked me on the head as I pushed up against the window frame for leverage in order to drill the holes in the molding to secure the L brackets. I found myself tangled in the window treatment cording, and the drill kept slipping off the screw, relentlessly punching Phillips head-shaped dents in my fingers. My arms fell asleep, because all this was happening above my head. I could see the Channel 9 news sound bite: "A local forty-three-year-old Northwood woman was found dead on her driveway after allegedly falling out a third-story window. Police are ruling out foul play, as the woman was found half-naked, with puncture wounds in her hands and a cordless drill by her side. Details at eleven."

In the end, I got the window treatments up, but the fight between woman and power tool was a draw. Brian came home from the gym and was blindsided to find the woman he left peacefully pinning fabric now a banshee woman sweating, pacing, and ranting. I'm sure he wondered if at any minute my head would spin and I'd spew pea soup. He stood frozen and wide-eyed as I ranted and screamed first about what an asshole my drill had been through the treatment-mounting project, then to how I knew I was now completely out of control. Within minutes, I ended up in a puddle of tears. Steroids: 1. Tracy: 0. When I took a moment to breathe and calm down, he suggested I have a little quiet time. I totally needed a time-out. And a couple of Xanax. And a margarita. Not necessarily in that order.

OK, so back to the support group. The social worker brought up the biggies. Maybe she did this every time. Maybe everyone feels what I was feeling, so she initiated the same topics over and again at each month's meeting, but whatever the reason, I was able to validate that I wasn't alone. Hearing other people say things that could have come directly from my mouth was intense. And I realized that I had become "the crier" at the meeting.

I have NEVER been a real crier for my own sake. Yes, I may well up and sniffle at hokey commercials, chick movies, and the proud moments of my life. I may cry as a patient cries in front of me and needs support, but crying has never really been an outlet for me. That was for other people, people who were more dramatic or had much worse things going on in their lives. When I was diagnosed, I didn't cry. I had to pay attention, listen, and plan.

Sure, once in a while, I strategically placed a cathartic bawl-fest into my repertoire when the right circumstances presented themselves. For example: When I was told I had Stage III cancer and not Stage IV, or when I heard Martina McBride's newly released "I'm Gonna Love You Through It" about a woman newly diagnosed with cancer. Those times? *Holy cow* did I bawl. But, for reasons beyond my comprehension, I'd now arrived at a new stage and level of release that only crying could satisfy. I somehow broke the seal for crying like a beer drinker's first pee at a bonfire. Once that seal is broken, you can't fight the urge to do it often . . . and shamelessly.

I didn't cry ALL the time, but the frequency was elevated from "rarely" to "often." I tried not to let it overcome me unless I was with someone with whom I felt safe, and I often cried alone just to get it out. Yet it was uncomfortable and still unfamiliar. I didn't recognize this blubbering idiot. *Who is she and how do I get the old Tracy back?*

At the meeting, it became clearer. Perhaps all of the drugs, toxins, and chemicals were wreaking havoc on my body, which increased my vulnerability and broke down my strength. That was certainly a possibility. However, when I asked, "Why do I cry now?", the answer was, "Because it is time."

I believe that each and every woman diagnosed with breast cancer is faced with a time when she realizes that she is no longer where – and maybe even who – she was before. For some, it becomes evident that they can no longer brush things under the rug and act as though they haven't had a life-changing experience. For others, it is surreal and very personal, and they reach out to only a few, if any, to share what they go through. It was a gradual realization for me. I was determined not to let this wretched disease alter me or take over my life or make me feel any different, but cancer is a game changer. Accepting that it *does* change the game sucks.

One woman's tipping point may be her final chemo. She might never have cried over the diagnosis; she might have gone through treatment strong, losing her hair, carrying on life fairly normally, until the day of her final chemo treatment, where she cries through the entire procedure. Another's might be in the second week of daily radiation, when she realizes that she is expected to absorb this time-consuming treatment disruption into her day but isn't given (and perhaps doesn't ask for) any slack, because she makes it all look so seamless and easy. Others continue and will always suffer in silence. Different things tip the scales for different people. We all have "our time," and we all cope differently.

Elizabeth Kübler-Ross describes five stages of dealing with grief. We all pass through each phase, even if for a short time, when dealing with personal change or trauma, as well as with death and dying. These stages are: denial, anger, bargaining, depression, and acceptance. I wasn't sure I could pinpoint which stages I'd been through and what the associated behavior was. I mainly felt that I went straight to acceptance. I mean really, I couldn't stop my diagnosis of cancer, it was what it was, so I might as well get on with it and look forward and keep a great attitude, right? Well, sort of right.

As I mentioned earlier, the second call I made was to my counselor, a woman who saw me through a difficult divorce. I had made her aware of my diagnosis shortly after I found out myself. But I knew I needed to experience the challenges of treatment firsthand, and we had left it that I would call her if I needed her. I knew that now, I needed her.

I called because I was crying so often. I realized that I needed to talk through some of what I was now feeling with someone who knew me, someone with whom I felt safe, someone who was not related to me. When we talked – well, I talked mostly – she reflected back to me a surprising fact: I was angry. Because I believe that everything happens for a reason, I am rather quick to accept and move on. I don't let myself sit in the anger. I feel yucky there. But if you don't sit in it, experience it, be "one" with the anger, you can't move *through* it. If you can't move through it, you are stuck. I was stuck. She told me that I needed to acknowledge it, and it was OK to be mad. So, I embraced the anger. *Hello. My name is Tracy, and I am ANGRY that I got cancer in the midst of an otherwise great life. There. Take that!*

Maybe a result of not letting myself be angry led to me holding in feelings, and then, when the dam broke, it all came out in the form of uncontrollable tears. Maybe it was that and the drugs, compounded by fatigue. I don't know exactly why, but it was my time to cry. Admitting that I was angry, then crying as a release, helped.

On Thursday, January 19, I had my last round of chemotherapy. I wanted to grab a tiara or crown, wear boas, eyebrows, and stilettos to celebrate . . . but the reality of the last treatment's significance hadn't hit me because it still felt so routine. I would, I hoped, have my last weekend of pain, narcotics, and steroids. And perhaps I could cut back on my meds and I'd soon feel a little love with the hair re-growth. I was SO not feelin' the love now. Also, along the lines of hair, I realized I missed nose hair, too. In cold weather, if the ole nose got runny, I had no little nasal follicular friends to hold it IN. Glamorous, huh? And because I want to you continue to read on, I won't expound on that visual any longer. You're welcome.

Once this modality of treatment was done, I would be almost halfway to the end. In the remainder of time ahead, I would try to give myself a break with responsibilities. I heard it takes a YEAR after chemo to recover to a point where a person feels close to the old normal. In both work and life, I would try not to push myself too hard. I would remain appreciative, stay positive, and always be thankful for all of the ways people helped. The game may have changed, but I had a strategy to win.

CHAPTER NINETEEN

The Term Paper

Saturday, January 21, 2012

DO YOU EVER recall a time in school where you were assigned a ten-page paper on a subject that bored you to tears? All the research, time, and organization you had to put in to finish it meant you had to kiss your weekends goodbye for a month. Unlike today, when I was in high school and college, computers weren't a household item, and rough drafts were done the "old-fashioned" way – on lined notebook paper. Back then, there was no such thing as a neat edit. There was no highlighting the area, tapping a quick "control x," then "control v," and voila! Edit done. No, edits looked more like scribbles, with big Xs or parentheses that surrounded the information that needed to be cut or moved. Multiple arrows, numbers, and stars polluted the margins.

Once said "editing" was done, the next task was to translate these hieroglyphics into a final, typed copy. For me, it was often like deciphering a treasure map. (Pass through the seven levels of the Candy Cane forest, then through the sea of swirly twirly gum drops, then walk through the Lincoln Tunnel . . . .) It was all-consuming, to say the least. So, picture the anticipation as the hours of research, writing, editing are all winding down. As you come down the home stretch, you are finally typing it all out. It's a work of art – double spaced, complete with footnotes, page numbers, and one-inch margins. But wait. Hang on a second! As you type it out, you realize that the thirteen pages of handwritten work yield only a mere four-and-a-half pages of double-spaced typing! *What? Say it ain't so! You have GOT to be KIDDING me!* The realization that you were only halfway done, when you thought you were ready to put that bad boy to bed, was THE worst. Those feelings of despair, resentment, and defeat were overwhelming as you tried to figure out how you would fill the next five-and-a-half pages, especially when you thought you had covered everything and there couldn't possibly be anything left to add. Your choices were: (1) accept it as was, turn it in, and take your chances with the grade, or (2) embrace it, be creative, and move forward. The first choice really wasn't an option. So back you went to look for more information in places that you didn't think to look before. You searched to come up with creative ways to improve what you had in order to transform the final paper into a work of art.

This particular week, the paper-writing experience reared its ugly head in my life journey, in the form of a number of frustrations, and, ultimately, a work of art. I shall explain.

At my second-to-last treatment, my oncologist asked me how I was going to "celebrate" the fact that I had finished chemotherapy. After all, it was a milestone. A big one, worth celebrating. I agreed. Of the four major pieces of this journey (mastectomy/surgery, chemotherapy, radiation therapy, and, finally, reconstructive surgery), I was about to finish my second, and probably the worst, "leg" of this trip. It did, in fact, deserve celebration. A few things went through my mind. One was that I had not yet had the opportunity to have any sort of "party" at my house since I'd moved in almost two years previously. I love to entertain. Having a reason to celebrate, being surrounded by those who knew what I was going through would make me feel good. I set a date.

On the last day of chemo, I dressed up. OK, I'll tell you 'cause I know you're dying to know – it's all about the outfit. Purple top, black leggings, a gold-and-purple headscarf, and my all-out, black, peep-toe, four-and-a-half-inch Coach heels from Vegas! I was ready to tackle this last dose of chemo head on! I went in and received the proper amount of acknowledgement for the shoes, but the overall experience wasn't what I thought it would be.

In my mind, this day was monumental – I no longer had to live in two-week increments and ride the rollercoaster of pain and fatigue! No more poison being pumped into my veins, no more feeling great just in time to be hit again with the next round. But, surprisingly, the day played out quite normally. There was nothing to separate it out as the "Last Treatment" – no balloons, no plastic tiara, no cake, no streamers, no blowy noisemaker things that unroll as you blow them. No fanfare. It was exactly what I had experienced every other week: the wonderful comfort of those I love around me . . . with the added bonus of "Boom Boom," the pet therapy greyhound. As sweet as he was, he didn't even give me a farewell lick to say, "best of luck" or a throw me a melancholy wayward greyhound glance as he was led away to the next patient. And my foot-rub lady, Diane, for the first time in eight visits, didn't come in.

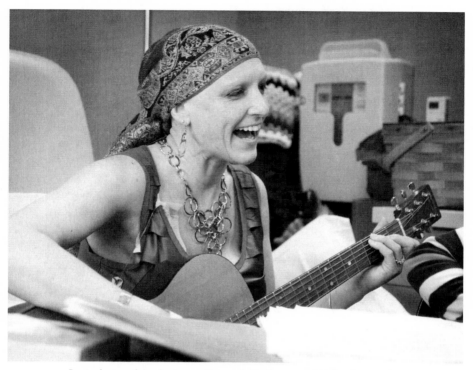

Last chemo day playing guitar and singing to make the time go by

However, I brought my guitar in again, and my girlfriend Frieda brought hers, too. We sang and played together, which passed the time very quickly. My mom and Brian had come with me that day, and Jody and my friend Carol, a veteran breast cancer survivor, stopped in to acknowledge the big day. Although everyone who visited made mention of it being the last time, by and large, it felt the same. At the end, the IV pump beeped to alarm us that it was all done, and nurse came in, unhooked me, flushed my line, and it was over.

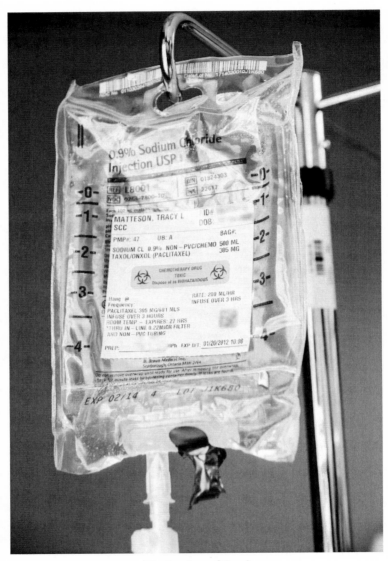

The last bag of Taxol

The rest of us sat there for a bit as we wrapped up the afternoon, wondering if maybe there was more. *Or, maybe I didn't want to leave.* I sat there thinking, I need it to sink in that this is the last dose of chemo. I needed to believe and acknowledge it, because if I didn't, maybe that really meant that I didn't believe it was really over. *Am I thinking it might come back? Is that why I didn't order the party hats? What if the fact that I'm not making this day a big deal means that I don't believe the cancer is really gone and that I will be back in this chair again?* I couldn't put any thought into that negativity. That was not me. So, I knew that somehow, I needed to acknowledge that chemo was done. Over. Finished. And that I would NOT in fact, be sitting in that chair again. I concentrated on the party I would be having a week from that day.

That night, as Brian and I raided the fridge for leftovers, I silently wished that there had been a special dinner waiting, a bottle of wine or champagne (even though I knew I shouldn't drink it) or perhaps even flowers. It would have felt like someone, aside from me, could appreciate to the same degree how significant that last chemo treatment was. I wanted something to be different that night to acknowledge that this WAS the last treatment. But I didn't communicate that to anyone. I played it cool and didn't make it a big deal. I didn't lay out what I wanted my evening to look like to anyone, and I now regretted it. On the outside, I had made it seem like just another day and that I was just glad to have it behind me. Cue the strong, glad-it's-over, good-riddance-to-chemo face.

On the inside, I had expected that it would be as big for everyone around me as it was for me, and that would be cause for a huge celebration. I felt like that person who says, "Whatever you do, DON'T throw me a surprise party," then suspects at every turn she'll walk into a room of people yelling, "SURPRISE!" But I hadn't said anything to anyone. Damn my bravery, nonchalantness (I made that word up), and silence. It bit me in the ass on this one.

I mentioned to my sister shortly after that I had secretly hoped someone would have known the extent to which that last chemo was significant to me. She responded with something that I never fully appreciated until that moment. She said, "The one thing that a cancer patient doesn't realize is that maybe for the first time, her family doesn't understand what she's going through." What a reality check. I had stepped outside of a life where everyone close to me knew the ins and outs of my needs. My family knows when I am hurting, when something is on my mind, or, as my intuitive mother says, when "something just isn't right," by my tone of voice or body language. They could relate to a hard day filled with running around crazy, or, as had happened recently, the stresses of trying to get Christmas shopping done for everyone when I had low energy. So, it seemed normal that they would understand the intensity of my needs as I dealt with cancer, too. But how would they? They could empathize and support (and I was blessed with how well they did both of these things), but unless they'd experienced it themselves, or I was specific with my communication, they couldn't know what I was feeling.

On this monumental day, because I couldn't verbalize exactly what I needed, each family member thought I'd be celebrating in a quiet and reflective way (which you would think may have sent up a flag, 'cause I'm not usually a "quiet" type of person), and, in fairness, I did say that my "celebration" would be the party I had planned. I found out that my Mom had been chomping at the bit to bring over dinner, because she really DID get it and wanted to make the night special for me. But instead, she didn't want to intrude on this reflective and perhaps emotional night for me. Everyone showed compassion by following my lead when it came to supporting me. They waited patiently for me to reach out so as not to be intrusive – which had been *exactly* how I wanted it.

But I didn't make a move. And now, I stood knocking on the door of "chemo finality" in my party dress, heels, and makeup, with a huge smile and a bottle of wine, ready to PARTY, but when invited to go in, I found everyone in jeans and flannel PJs sipping their tea, snuggled up under blankets, watching documentaries. No one can read my mind. This was the first time I wished they could have.

Celebrations aside, the weekend after my last treatment was better than any of my previous recovery times. Friday, due to the pre-med IV steroids the day before, I had the strength and energy of ten women and went on a mad cleaning spree, where I went from room to room to room cleaning and scrubbing and wiping things down. I went from vacuuming crumbs in cabinets to hanging up pictures that had been sitting on the floor, four feet below where they should be. Brian watched me flying from here to there when he came home from work on Friday and said, "Um, you're scaring me a little."

I wanted to be able to recoup and not look around at what needed to be done. Unfortunately, trying to settle down was hard and led into a restless night of sleep (the steroids kept me up as well), because my brain wouldn't shut down as it continued to make mental lists of what else I could clean. (My car could use a good vacuuming . . . and I never did get to the windowsills . . . .) I lay in bed, mind spinning, as the intermittent hot flashes brought me restlessly into Saturday morning. This was usually the morning I wanted to ball up into the fetal position from the head to toe because of the pain and aches. But that Saturday morning, although I was not pain free, my pain without the Neulasta shot was cut by half. I still ached, but mostly from the waist down and not nearly as intensely. I was tired and let myself rest for the weekend in my freshly cleaned house. Monday, I began my next step.

On Monday, Brian and I met my radiation oncologist, who was the perfect complement to the cancer center oncology team. He was personable, allowed me to ask questions, smiled, was light hearted, and wasn't in the least bit rushed. He set up my "mapping" appointment for Monday, February 13. At that time, I would have a CT scan, then tattoos (three freckle-sized dots) would be placed to align me correctly for the radiation therapy (XRT). I had a month off before I would start another "leg" of treatment.

He confirmed that it would be a good idea for me to see my plastic surgeon in Boston on Wednesday to see if she would advise having any saline taken *out* of my expanders. Sometimes, the unaffected expander/breast on the opposite side of treatment is in the direct line of the radiation beams and needs to be deflated to clear that path. Sometimes, the plastic surgeons prefer preemptive deflation to be safe. I looked forward to that visit, because I would find out a bit find more out about my final surgery plan, and I hoped to nail down a more specific timeline as far as next steps went, relating to my reconstruction.

I left the appointment with this new doctor, feeling pleased and confident yet again with my oncology team. He had answered all of my questions and gave me a detailed description of what I could expect. It felt good to leave a doctor's office thinking, "This is someone I would enjoy spending time with in a non-medical social situation." The providers were closer to my age these days, and their energy and personalities shone through in their daily duties. I left feeling that had just added another great player to my team.

Fast forward two days. I headed to Boston with Frieda to see my plastic surgeon. She was coming full circle with the doctor's visits, as she had also accompanied me to my first all-day appointment in Boston when I was first diagnosed. Again, I went in prepared, with my notebook and a list of questions.

The first and most important question was, how long after the radiation treatment would I need to heal before I had my final surgery? I had my timeline all mapped out in my head. Mastectomy in September: check. Chemo from October to January: check. Radiation from February through beginning of April: check. Final plastic surgery end of May: check. Out mowing my own lawn, feeling good, doing all the things I used to do by the fourth of July . . . MAYBE even feeling good in a bathing suit! I also had more immediate questions: Did I need to have anything more done with the expanders? Was I all set, or did I need to have any more saline put in or taken out to get back to my pre-mastectomy size? How did things look now? What about the biopsy scar and my port?

Frieda and I went into the exam room. I changed into my gown, and we waited. My plastic surgeon came in, and we exchanged pleasantries . . . but that is where any form of pleasant ended for me. She took a look at my expanders and did say that everything looked good and appeared to be well healed. She asked where I was in my overall treatment, and I told her that I was going to have the "mapping" for the XRT on February 13 and wanted to try to coordinate in case she felt that I needed to have my size altered for treatment. She said no.

She also felt that the expanders were the right size and that I didn't need anything more injected, so unless the XRT people requested that I need to have saline taken out for treatment, she was all done with me until after the XRT. This led to the perfect segue into my most important question. I asked her point blank how long before the finish line, the end point, the boobie prize. (I didn't really ask her that way.) She said that she would meet up with me for a follow-up appointment six to eight weeks after I was done with the XRT, but that the actual surgery couldn't be done for at LEAST three to six *months* after treatment was over. My brain shut off. *What? Back the truck up for a second here. Did she just say three to six MONTHS after I finish radiation? Does she know that is WAY outside of my timeline? Did she miss the memo that stated I was expecting to be bathing-suit ready by July?* I sat there having an out of body experience. It was just like the day my surgical oncologist told me that I needed a mastectomy instead of a lumpectomy. I wanted to cry on the spot. Charlie Brown's teacher entered the room again, and all I heard was "mwa mmwaa wa waaa" as I tried to shuffle this new timeline around in my head. One by one, all of the organized questions I had been ready to ask started to fall away. Frieda reached for my notebook and took over, asking the questions that I couldn't articulate, like, "What is the reason we need to wait such a long time?" and "When should the port be removed?"

When I could feel myself coming back into my body, I could barely breathe an audible word but managed to get out, "I am feeling very out of control right now. I need more information in order to grasp things; can we please go over a little bit about my surgery? How long will it take and what can I expect?" I was trying desperately to find my happy place.

She looked at me and said, "I'm not going to go over that with you now. It is too early. I need to see you after your radiation to see how things look first, and then we will formulate a plan."

Access denied. No entry. Please reverse direction. Any iota of control I had was slipping through my fingertips. *What? She isn't even going to humor me through this? She's shutting me down? What about the patient's right to know? What about compassion? What about explaining why she doesn't want to talk about it? Does she have too many patients who have things go wrong during radiation and she doesn't want to get my hopes up or scare me with statistics? Well, what scares me is not knowing! Is there a group of patients out there who don't do well with radiation due to some common denominator that I may have? What is it? Eating too many bananas? A similar body type or bust size to mine? Was it the Stage III cancer patients who had undergone chemo and didn't do well?*

I knew I wanted to verbalize questions, and I knew that if I didn't say something in response to this general dismissal soon, I might totally lose my chance. I was like Ralphie, the little boy on *A Christmas Story* whose mind goes blank when he sits on Santa's lap. (Football? What's a football?) I was about to be pushed down that slide, when I snapped back into some form of reality and was able to say, "OK then, what could go wrong with the radiation that would change the surgical reconstruction plan? Hypothetically, when I come back to see you, best-case scenario, you will look at me and say, "You've healed well; let's plan a date for surgery and proceed as planned." (That would mean expanders out, implants in.) "If THAT does not happen, what are the other possible things that you would say? What is Plan B?"

It was then that I realized that the effects of radiation may have more of an impact on my final surgery than I had thought. Yes, the initial radiation oncologists I saw months ago told me there was a small chance that XRT could hurt implants if they were put in at the same time as the mastectomy. I knew this and understood that I needed to do whatever would give me the best chance at looking "normal" after reconstruction. But it wasn't until now that I was hearing more of the details or risks of how XRT could really complicate things. Was it scary and a bit unnerving? Sure. But did I want to know and understand? Absolutely. She explained that if there was "too much damage" and my pectoral muscle wouldn't support the implant, they might have to move muscle from my back to my chest. That would be a totally different reconstruction than what I hoped to have. But that was as much as she said, and she reiterated that we really just needed to see what things looked like after radiation before we could formulate any sort of real plan. That left me feeling dissatisfied, as if I had only just scratched the surface of questions.

Frieda asked to see before-and-after pictures. Buzzer sounded! Nope. Sorry. Apparently, she needed to "update her book" and really didn't have anything that could fairly represent a woman who'd had a mastectomy, chemo, radiation, and then implants. *Really? Wasn't I referred to her because she was one of Boston's best plastic surgeons? And she didn't have anything she could show me?* At that point, even though she sat in front of me and quietly waited for the next question, no matter what we asked, it felt as though we got short, curt answers. ("Should I have the port taken out?" "Yes, that needs to be out because it will be in my way." You get the gist.). I felt she responded with the minimum answers in order to discourage more questions, and I was ready to get the hell outta Dodge. Utterly frustrating. That ended my appointment. I had more questions now than when I first came in.

After she left, Frieda looked at me and said, "What are you feeling? What's going on?" I was tearing up, feeling completely out of control, very dismissed. I needed time to process. Experiencing a doctor visit minus the warm fuzzies, plus being treated with a dismissive demeanor didn't help me at all. But I recalled that she had been very matter-of – fact when I met her for the first time, too.

Frieda was able to lay it out for me. She said, "It may have felt as though this doctor did not have much of a warm personality today, but she *undersells* and will *overdeliver*. She doesn't want your expectations to be too high, so that when she *does do* a great job, it will be even better." I had to run with the fact that she has a great reputation and is known to produce a fantastic final product. But now I was looking at October at the earliest for surgery. It left me frustrated and hollow, as if I'd just typed out my paper from the rough draft and found that I had only four pages and still had five to go, when I thought that I had at least at seven completed.

I went home and held it together until after dinner. Then, I did what an old friend always told me I needed to do more. He used to tell me, "You need to get in touch with your inner bitch . . . and get mad." Oh, yeah. I went there. I got mad. And I cried. Hard. Can't-breathe-through-your-nose, eyes-swollen-almost-closed hard. I had been patient. I had rolled with treatment this far. I complained minimally, pushed forward, tried to communicate, and made the lemonade out of these lemons to the best of my ability. I had tried to keep the changes in my life and those around me to a minimum. So, I *didn't deserve* to be dismissed when

I needed information. I was *tired* of waiting. I wanted to be "normal" again (yes, I use that term loosely). I didn't want to walk by a mirror and not recognize that woman. I wanted to put on mascara, and a bra, and put gel in my hair. It all came flooding over me. Brian sat next to me, listened helplessly, handed me Kleenex, rubbed my back, and acknowledged my frustration. There wasn't a catch phrase I was looking for to make me "feel better." I just needed to get it OUT. And that I did. It was a good, cleansing release.

But poor Donald heard me from upstairs, and as I was trying to pull it together, he descended from the study, his chin quivering, tears welled up in his eyes, unable to say anything. I hadn't realized that he could hear me. When I asked him what was wrong, he simply said, "You're crying," as he tried to be brave and wipe away the tears. It shook him up. I had to gather myself to tell him that I was OK, that I was frustrated with things at this very moment, and I was trying to process and accept some new information and needed to let it out instead of keep it in. Dealing with frustration is an ever-changing process. I have now learned that getting in touch with my inner bitch leads me to crying it out, which feels good, but I perhaps I need to control when and where that happens, and the kids should be completely out of earshot. Lesson number 834 in this journey, filed away.

I had a tumultuous week for sure. But, I'd planned the "Halfway There" party . . . the first party I'd have in my new house. I invited a Silpada jewelry rep and a Party Lite Candle rep to come. Although I didn't want to make it about the jewelry or candles, I thought that this way, people could have nice things to look at while I mingled and greeted people at the door and tried to do some hostess duties. I made it about me. I served pink drinks (which, due to an untimely snowstorm, were not consumed to the extent that I thought they might be), appetizers, and a houseful of warmth, love, and laughter. I dressed in pink and was able to greet and embrace everyone as they came through the door.

This is the time in treatment where patients tend to feel deserted . . . the waiting, the in-between, the lull. But that night, I felt anything but deserted. I felt the love. The support and the joy. The feelings of frustration and anger from just twenty-four hours before were gone. The presence of these people at this party was exactly what I needed.

Have you ever bought a new car and then noticed how many others like yours are on the road? Or gotten pregnant and then realized that you could pick a woman in her first trimester out of a crowd? It's like that with cancer, too. I was walking through Target, and a woman stopped me and asked me "my story." She showed me her hair and said, "One year of growth." My scarves and naked hairless face was telling, but thankfully, it didn't scare off other survivors. I also realized how many other people had been put into my life to get me through this. They came up to me and said all sorts of things – they'd been there, they were two years cancer free, they didn't have nipples and wanted to show me their scars (maybe not at Target!), did I want someone to talk to (because they always seemed to know someone who'd been in a similar situation and who had a bright attitude and would be a good person to talk to). They came out of the woodwork. I'd never seen them before, but they seemed to present themselves when I needed them most. I just had to be watching for them.

So what was next? Where was I now? Well, for starters, I was inches from my mirror at every opportunity, watching closely as the fine new white hair came in on my head. I expected it to be prickly, like hair that has been shaved. But it wasn't. It was new, soft, and fine, and yes, all snow white. I was in a holding pattern now with my treatment as I healed and let the chemo work its magic and give my body a rest from all the toxins. I tried to seek some normalcy as I didn't feel the pressure of doctor's appointments every week. I still had questions, but I'd just call to get my answers. I was given a half-dozen phone numbers of people to call that perhaps I would get around to. I was overwhelmed at the thought of being thrown back into the workplace and parenting life, but each day, as I got another good day behind me, it seemed less daunting. I still got tired and suffered from "chemo brain" (where I couldn't find the right word or could multi-task only eight things and not twelve), so I worked from home early in the morning when I was feeling well, and then in the evening when I got my second wind. I did yoga and planned to exercise, tone up, and ask for help when I needed it.

My ten-page "cancer paper" has had a lot of editing. There are scribbles in the margins (things I didn't do well), there are paragraphs written with passion (things I did do well), and I thought I was closer to completion than I found I actually was. But the condensed five pages I wrote and experienced are solid. And full of lessons. And I was OK with being only halfway done. The due date for completion was pushed out to early to mid-fall. There was a lot more to write. But until then, I'd enjoy the good days and not get discouraged. Life was good.

CHAPTER TWENTY

Just Call Me Buffy

Sunday, February 12, 2012

THESE DAYS, WHEN we hear the name "Buffy," the thought of a young blonde with impractical running shoes (God love her!) who slays vampires and executes all things evil comes to mind for many people. I could never embrace the fact that the name "Buffy" was picked for a Vampire Slayer because, for me, the name "Buffy" represented a much different person. When I was a kid, *Sesame Street* occasionally guest-starred a Native American named Buffy. She had long, dark hair occasionally adorned with feathers, dark brown eyes, and beautiful skin. I was mesmerized by her natural beauty.

When my sister and I were young and played together, we'd start off an afternoon imagination adventure by picking out what and who we were going to be. Anna and I would take turns playing Buffy. I had short, blonde hair and blue eyes, but when it was my turn to be Buffy, I went through a slight transformation. Minus the buckskin dress, moccasins, and feather headdresses, I would sometimes put a dark tee shirt over my head, then pull it back up over my face and wear it inside-out with the neck of the shirt on my hairline (with the body of the shirt falling down my back) in lieu of long black hair. Naturally, this was all it took to ultimately transform me into a natural Native American beauty – a little fake tee-shirt hair, imagination, and attitude. Who'd have thought hair might make that much of a difference in my self-perception?

Here's my take on that.

It was a little past three weeks since my last chemo. On the day that I *would have* had my chemo, I celebrated with Frieda and Jody by having dinner in Portsmouth. It was a wonderfully intimate celebration, and it felt nice, not only because was it a fun night out, but also because I was actually feeling *good* . . . and I knew that I wasn't about to go into a weekend of feeling lousy. I continued to get stronger every day. The month before, I was overwhelmed, because after chemo, I wouldn't be doing anything active to fight the recurrence of cancer. I was afraid I'd be thrown back into the "she's good to go now" bucket, and the hectic, crazy life of juggling everything would resume. I thought, "How on earth will I be able to manage it all?" What I didn't fully comprehend was that my body was still hopped up on chemo and other drugs that made me vulnerable and void of strength, both mental and physical.

So, I went back to working more normal hours and was able to drive hither and yon for kid stuff, and although there were days where I had to stop and take a quick nap, I was feeling much better. The challenge was that I needed to be out among people . . . no longer did I feel justified in hiding in the safety of my home because I didn't feel quite up to par. I started wearing "dress casual" attire for work. At home, Garwood (my black lab) didn't seem to mind that I wore exercise clothes, sweats, or comfy clothes, with an ugly (but practical) cap on my head to keep warm. My home standard didn't include makeup or, frankly, sometimes even a shower first thing in the morning. Naturally, it wouldn't make sense to shower in case I got the sudden urge to exercise. (Admittedly, the yoga routines I was doing rarely worked up a sweat unless I experienced a hot flash, but it *could* happen, right?)

During home days, I aimed to tip the "presentable scale" slightly, so that in case the UPS truck stopped by with a package, I wouldn't scare the delivery person when I opened the door. OK, yes, seeing that in black and white, I realize that the bar had been significantly lowered. But getting ready to go out anywhere took SO much time and effort. I've always been a pretty low-maintenance gal. I've always kept my hair short so I don't need a brush or blow-drier . . . all I have to do is dip into a tiny bit of hair gel, scrunch it in, and I'm good to go. I wear minimal makeup and concentrate more on matching accessories with my outfit. I try to keep it simple.

I embraced the fact that I was now in a state of temporary, post-chemo-appearance limbo. I was down to two eyelashes on each upper eyelid. I had about ten eyebrow hairs over my right eye and maybe double that over my left eye, which generally rendered my facial expression as quizzical. (I guess that's better than surprised or angry.) The money I saved on mascara was now going toward false eyelashes. Since I was feeling a bit better, I now had energy and interest in exploring new and more exciting follicular options.

Cue "Samantha the Lash Lady." I happened to meet her on a night where I was sporting my Vegas showgirl lashes, and she commented on them. After chatting a bit, I found out that she too had breast cancer and was only a year or so into the survivor category. She gave me her number and told me that she would be happy to put on lashes that would last longer than just the day. This sounded like a fantastic idea, because I fought with my false lashes. Samantha was an energetic woman from Britain who described herself, in jest, as "extra." (I believe that is loosely translated as "eccentric.") I imagined what it would be like to have lashes that didn't jab into my eyeballs for eight consecutive hours due to lopsided application, and decided to call her to make an appointment.

I saw her one Friday. Samantha had invited me to come for lunch since I was coming straight from work. I arrived and we had a wonderful meal, then she showed me around and introduced me to her husband, who was working at home. After lunch, she went to work on me, applying little clumps of lashes to my lids with what looked like tar. I found out that she also did makeovers. She applied my makeup and topped it off by asking if I wanted to see her wig. I said sure. Now, before her treatment, Samantha had beautiful, shoulder-length, red ringlets. They were gorgeous! Her hair was now growing out as curly as ever, in the same color, and was four or five inches long and just as soft and stunning. But when she was going through treatment and had no hair, she looked into wigs and decided on a straight, long, red-haired wig. Why not? It was just as striking as her own hair.

She offered to let me borrow it.

You may recall the adventures of buying my first wig. It was when I still had hair, and my hairdresser Lisa and I tried our hardest to find a wig that was most like my natural hair – I just wanted to look like *me* (which I now realize was my downfall). We went with the one that matched the color of my hair the closest, and Lisa trimmed it up to make it a little sassier. But as many times as I put it on to give it a whirl, I couldn't seem to warm up to it. I just didn't love it. The wig and I had serious bonding issues. It was just different enough from my old style that it looked fake. So, when Samantha offered me a LONG, RED-HAIRED wig, I thought, "Well this is the most ridiculous thing I've ever heard of, but why not try it? What do I have to lose?"

I have *never* had long hair. Ever. I have tried a number of times to grow it out, at which time I made appointments with Lisa every three weeks to shape it, because the curl goes out of control. But ultimately, I get it about two to three inches long, and can't stand it, and we cut it off, wondering why I ever tried to grow it in the first place.

Samantha showed me how to put her wig on, and she pointed me to a mirror. With my new lashes and very natural makeup, I really liked what I saw! And I was shocked at how much I looked like my oldest daughter, Samantha! It was a new-looking me . . . I had been transformed on the outside to an adult version of Buffy. Instead of an inside-out tee shirt hanging down my back, I had beautiful red tresses that convinced me that normalcy wasn't that far-fetched or far off. I looked totally different, but soft and pretty, and I certainly didn't look like someone going through treatment for cancer. As much as I had been used to my short hair, I realized that the same rule applied to any drastic change in my hair as it did to the drastic change in my (previous) breasts – it didn't (they don't) define who I am. Just because I have always had short hair didn't mean that I wouldn't be who I am with long(er) hair. At that point I thought, Why not?

I said yes, I'd love to borrow the wig.

Practically speaking, I found advantages to wearing one. I am a matchy-matchy person. I like to coordinate my outfits and accessories. Some days, I got all dressed, and then realized I didn't have a headscarf that matched anything I had on. It was frustrating. Those were the days that I just plain wanted hair. (Have you ever noticed that hair matches everything?) I found that flipping on a wig was less time consuming than trying to coordinate just one more thing – brushing time included. And secondly, I have to admit that watching a family member, co-worker, or friend experience the shock factor when I casually walked in was SO FUN!

Example: I had to meet the new accountant at work one Saturday morning. The previous chairman would also be there to introduce me to her. I pulled up in my car, which he recognized, but when I walked to the locked building and saw him at the top of the steps, he looked at me and walked back into the office instead of helping me unlock the door. Once I was in, I bounded up the stairs and into the office, where I said, "Well, that wasn't very nice leaving me out in the cold. Don't you recognize me?" He stared silently at me with that "I think I know you" expression until it clicked! He kept saying, "Oh my God! I can't believe it's you! You look so different! Look at you!" The moment of realization was priceless.

My family reacted in a similar way. I sent a picture to my daughter Samantha right after I had the makeover. Her friend Abby had her phone and saw the picture come up. She said, "Who's that?" Samantha looked at it and said, "I don't know." She finally made the connection when she saw my text accompanying it, and she texted me her shocked reaction, "Mom! OMG! I didn't even recognize you!" And Donald . . . he came up the basement stairs and saw me and kept walking with his eyes as wide as saucers and his mouth open. When he could finally think of something to say, he uttered, "Are you going to wear that *all* the time?" That was a little more subtle than when Abigail took one look at me and said, "It's so not you." To which I responded, "It is today!" And when I walked into my mother's and father's house, my mom looked at me and burst into laughter (in a supportive, "I-can't-believe-it!" kind of way), and my dad walked around the corner, saw me, and smiled his "Holy Cow!" smile.

I must say that I don't know how women with long hair do it. As much as I like the look, I don't like the feeling of hair in my face or over my eyes. Perhaps it was a genetic female thing, but I instinctively took to a foreign, hair-flipping motion that I previously had never even thought about. I was also aware of the tickling of individual strands of hair on my face and neck. But although it was distracting, I keep getting back to, "It's fun! And I am damn well ready for a little fun!" When I think about it, I hope I won't ever have (knock on wood) another time in my life to try out long hair. I mean, really, what other situation would drive a person to say, "I think I will change my hair color and length today," and not have people around her say, "Why would you do that?" At that time, I had a quarter-inch of white peach fuzz on my head, and I looked as if I had a ringside seat to the Chernobyl meltdown. That was the "why" for me – seriously, who could blame me?

So, I went to a wig bank in Dover and got another more conservative, yet equally as fun, chin-length wig. It was a little darker than my normal hair, had bangs so it wasn't in my eyes, and was closer to the familiar "Tracy" look we'd all been used to. BONUS: It was FUN!

Please note that the following information is worth filing away. There are "wig banks," where the American Cancer Society donates wigs to cancer patients FREE OF CHARGE! Yes, it's true! All you have to do is make a private appointment. They'll ask you to fill out a form after you state what type of cancer you have, and then they'll ask if they can contact you. Many of the wigs are made from REAL hair donated from the "beautiful lengths" drives, where people donate their hair like my friend Robyn did for me a few months beforehand. The natural-hair wigs can be flat-ironed or curled and treated like the real hair that they're made from.

I've read alarming statistics about the number of people expected to get cancer in the future, so I pass this information on in the hopes that anyone who loses hair from cancer knows that this is an option. Real-hair wigs normally cost upwards of 350 dollars. Free worked much better for my budget.

I found myself having many dreams that involved hair growth. I dreamt that when it came in, I looked like Sinead O'Connor. I looked "hair" up in my dream book. (Yes. I have a dream book.) It said, "Hair represents strength and virility. Combing the hair is to be attempting to untangle a particular attitude we may have. To have our hair cut is to be trying to create order in our lives. To be cutting someone else's hair may be to be curtailing an activity. To be bald in a dream is to perhaps recognize one's own intelligence." (From *The Complete Book of Dreams & Dreaming* by Pamela Ball, Arcturus Publishing Limited, 2003.) Unfortunately, it says nothing about *growing* hair. More than likely, I was just dreaming about it because I was thinking about it so often. But I ran with the bald theory, since my intelligence did need recognizing, and if I didn't recognize it, who would?

I felt blessed that I had this down time to have some fun, and I was reminded a little about what my schedule and life were like before cancer paid me a visit. I'd start my next series of treatments in another week or so. At that point, I would be back to the daily reminder that I didn't have my life entirely back quite yet. Since adding on an extra two hours to my day wasn't an option, I would have to find a way to incorporate a daily interruption for treatment into my routine with as minimal disruption to work, family, and taking care of myself as possible.

In this next phase, I could go forward with the options of scarves AND various hair choices. I could throw on my wig and assume the role of the adult counterpart of Buffy. But in the end, I knew – scarf, long hair, medium hair, or Chernobyl hair – I was still me, and every day, I found a little more positive attitude to prove it.

CHAPTER TWENTY-ONE

Chutes and Ladders

Saturday, February 25, 2012

R EMEMBER *CHUTES AND Ladders*? It's a fairly straightforward kid's board game with one hundred spaces, ten per row, where you roll a die, move your player, and do one of three things: (1) Stay where you are (boring!), (2) Go up a ladder, which brings you closer to the finish line, or (3) Go down a chute, which sets you back, closer to the start line. Most of the chutes and ladders are fairly short, so you get you slightly ahead or behind, which keeps the excitement and competition of the game on a pretty even keel.

But, to keep it interesting, there are two humdingers thrown in there. After you're all warmed up and sitting confidently on the third row, with one lucky roll of the die, you could possibly land on space number twenty-eight, the mother lode, the king of all ladders, the golden rung to the finish line that brings you not just up a row or two, but up to space eighty-four, on the *second to last row*. Oh. My. Gosh. It's *so* hard not to gloat or at least try to cover up the coy smile that says, "Ha ha! See ya, suckers!" (Which is *not* a recommended phrase to use when playing against younger kids, um, so I've heard.)

The trouble is, after you've been lucky enough to make that bee line to the top of the stepladder of satisfaction, you realize that although the finish line is only sixteen spaces away, four of those spaces are chutes! That leaves you with a one-in-four chance of plummeting back down with the commoners! As you sit atop your runged throne, you strategically anticipate where your next move could put you. Lightly kissing the die, you inaudibly whisper the desperate plea into your hand – "Anything but a three" – before releasing it to the board. A three would put you on space eighty-seven, the space that has been known to bring even the strongest of players to despair. If you were fortunate enough to climb the aforementioned "golden ladder" and showed even an ounce of boasting, hitting this space is the great equalizer, as you nose-dive down to space twenty-four, avoiding eye contact with your peers, who are nodding, thinking, "Uh huh, Who's doing that victory dance now?"

But the worst is when you have been biding your time methodically, patiently, and with calm assurance to get to the second-to-last row. Hitting space eighty-seven is utterly devastating. You are back at the bottom . . . all that hard work for naught. You had only thirteen spaces left to navigate through; now, you have seventy-six. It feels as if you will never get there.

I'd been playing a fair game and was making my way up the board, but this week, I was pretty sure that I hit my very own, personal "space eighty-seven."

Monday, February 13, began my next run of doctors' and treatment appointments. I enjoyed my month off. I had started exercising, eating better, and feeling more energy than I had in months. With a schedule void of one doctor's appointment after the next, life was even a little more familiar. But I knew that all good things must come to an end, so I was ready to tackle the next phase of this journey: radiation therapy.

On all accounts, I'd been told that the radiation phase was supposed to be easier than surgery or chemotherapy. The ups and downs wouldn't be as intense; fatigue might kick my butt or slow me down, but, I hoped, not incapacitate me. Friends I knew who'd been through radiation said they felt fatigue, but it was often hard to tell if it was from the effect of the therapy itself or from the extra effort and energy it took to juggle yet one more thing into an already packed day. Either way, I was aware of the effects, and I was ready.

On February 13, Brian and I went in for the first step of my radiation therapy: mapping. Mapping is the process of marking a patient with dot-sized tattoos so that at every daily appointment, the radiation technicians can carefully align a patient the exact same way so that the radiation hits very specific target areas. The process for determining placement is complex and methodical. It includes a team of professionals: radiation technicians, radiation oncologists, and even a physicist. There are simulators, 3-D images, and specific programs. And – bonus – it is painless.

I checked in with the same familiar wonderful staff that I had for my chemotherapy. A nurse led us to an exam room where I met my radiation oncologist, and we briefly talked to the doctor about the process. He was warm, assuring, and kind. I felt reassured.

Brian and I were then separated. I was directed to the ladies' waiting room, and he was directed to the men's waiting room area. I had been instructed to remove my clothing from the waist up and put on a johnny.

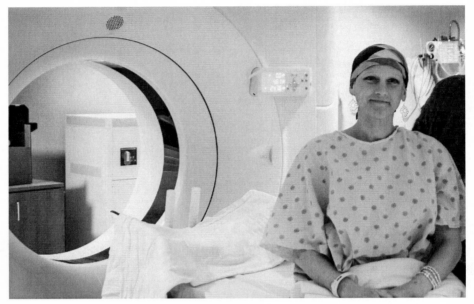

The CT machine for mapping

The wait was only a couple of minutes before we were brought into a room where there was a large machine that looked like a CT scanner. I lay down on a plank designed to move through a big circle, where the scan is simulated. I was covered with warm blankets, and the tech there assisted me with pulling my arms out of the gown. My head was turned to the left so that they could include the nodes near my right collarbone in the scan. Both of my arms were extended above my head. Brian snapped photos. At the point where they needed to expose my right side, the staff shuffled Brian out.

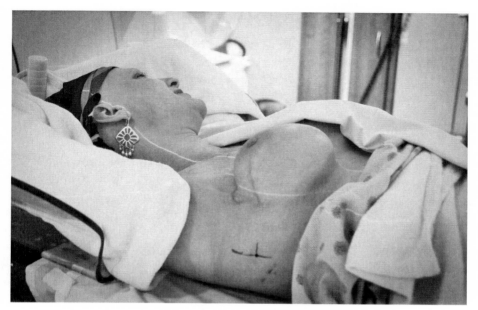

Lasers aligned to place markers

They kept my left side covered and exposed my right expander/breast. My doctor then appeared and marked me with a black Sharpie marker on both sides lateral to my expanders (on my ribcage), and then made two marks in my cleavage. Red laser beams that radiated from the ceiling and side of the scanner adorned various areas of my sides and chest. Tiny, sticky BBs were placed at the Sharpie marks. These spots were where the laser lines coincided. I was told to hold still as everyone left the room and the plank slowly moved me through the scanner and back a few times. I heard the whirr of the machine and a beep that sounded like my dishwasher does when it has finished its cycle. My arms went numb as I lay there as still as I could.

When I was pulled back out of the machine, I asked for Brian to come back so that he could continue taking pictures. I was very grateful for the respect for privacy, but I wanted to know what this looked like (for realsies!). I told them I was OK with him seeing me vulnerable and exposed, and it was important to me to have him capture what this process really looked like.

I'd had a mild level of anxiety going in for this piece of the journey. Normally, I ask a ton of questions, but I felt I might sound dumb if I asked questions like, "What does the machine look like?" "How long will it take?" and "What exactly is the process, and what can I expect?" Would they look at me like, "What are you? Five years old?" Did I really need to know the answers to those questions? Probably not. But was I wondering? Yes, I was. As a nurse, I never worked oncology, let alone a specialty area like radiation, so I had no idea of what to expect. Knowledge is power. I should have asked, and I know in my heart that they wouldn't have chastised or belittled me, but instead, I just put on my brave face and thought, "I'll learn as I go, and I'll document for others."

As I waited for Brain to return, I lay on the table complete with BBs, Sharpie marks, and an exposed breast. It was time to be tattooed for real. The radiation tech in the room dropped a single drop of ink on the four BB areas, then went back and said, "Bee sting." I felt the stings as the tattoos were being done. They hadn't told me it was OK to move my head so I couldn't watch or see any part of what she was doing – and she did all four so fast that they were done before Brian was back. He immediately started documenting what everything looked like. I was glad he did. I had experienced what it was like to lie there and have limited vision due to the position of my head and body, but I had no idea what it looked like or what was going on.

Similarly, when I was in nursing school, I never got to see a live birth. I'd sit and try to comfort laboring women for an eight-hour shift, and inevitably, I would need to leave right before anything crucial happened. The first live birth I experienced was when I gave birth to Samantha, only it was from the other "end," with a much different perspective! Seeing it and experiencing it were two different things. As I reviewed Brian's pictures, it was like seeing it all for the first time.

I got dressed, and another tech met me in the waiting area. She gave me a calendar printout of my schedule for the next three months, with times and places for my upcoming treatments. They were very conscious of patients' schedules and had asked me what time would work the best for me. I asked for a 2:30 pm slot so that I could work in the morning at the office and then leave for the day to have my radiation. I wanted to be careful not to overdo it. Something had to give in my daily routine so that radiation could fit in: work, family time, healing time, or personal time. A 2:30 pm slot seemed to be a good compromise for me not taking too much time from my work day, yet also not taking too much time from the other important areas of my life.

The schedule reflected that Tuesday would be my "sim" verification, where they would do a simulation of the actual treatment based on all the tattoos and marks to verify that everything was aligned and they weren't accidentally radiating my earlobe or something. They added in a little extra time just in case last-minute adjustments needed to be made. Then, Wednesday was to be the big day. Day one of twenty-eight total doses. The schedule was Monday through Friday, and they outlined a six-week schedule, factoring in "just in case" scenarios.

As it was laid out, the first week someone else was slotted for 2:30, but they juggled my times around a bit so that I could get started. Wednesday and Thursday, I had the same time slot, but Friday was different, too. I made appointments and scheduled projects and errands around these times. I needed to be flexible if I wanted this to be seamless, right? So, I was going with the flow.

When Tuesday arrived, I went to work and planned my day around my appointment. I was actually feeling a bit on the sassy side, because I had started to wear my mid-length wig to work. I headed to the cancer center with enough time to register yet not be too early. The ladies at the reception made the appropriate amount of fanfare and fuss over the wig. When I checked in, the receptionist said, "You're here for a visit with the doctor?" to which I replied, "No, I am here for my sim verification." She looked puzzled and said that her computer reflected a doctor's visit, but she would go right back and get it figured out for me. This conflict wasn't a good sign. She came back and said that the nurse was with another patient but would come right out and get me. That was all she knew.

Moments later, the nurse did come get me. Instead of heading to the changing room, I was ushered into an exam room. She sat me down and said, "The doctor wants to meet with you today to talk to you. You won't be having your sim verification. It has to do with your expanders." All I could do was utter, "Shit."

I was glad that no one was taking my vitals or that the room wasn't being monitored, because behind that closed door I was swearing like a sailor. *Come ON! How. Could. This. Be?* I had *specifically* asked questions to address concerns about the expanders and avoid any possible delays. Krikey! I even made a trip to Boston to be double sure no more saline needed to be added or taken out! The fact that I asked questions, planned, and did everything I could to ensure that things would go smoothly and they still *didn't* made me MENTAL!

Very early on, I had been told there was a chance that this would happen. But at my introduction appointment, the doctor said he thought that I would be fine and didn't see that my size would be a problem. I tried not to get worked up in the little exam room, but with every second that passed, the urge to run increased.

He came in with his handsome, sparkly smile and demeanor and asked how I was. I looked like a deer in the headlights; it took me a second to decide how to answer such a question. Did I go with the polite response: "I'm fine thanks, and how are you"? Or the real answer: "I'm on the edge, feeling way out of control, anxious, and seriously want to punch something"? I couldn't shoot the messenger, so I opted for mid-ground: "Well, I guess 'not so good,' because I'm here and not in the changing room." It came out more sarcastic than I had intended, but I'm pretty sure that the look on my face helped him understand it was the anxiety talking.

He responded right away. "No, you're fine; you're good, just a little setback." He went on to explain that because of the size of my expanders, the rays were aligned in such a way that, unfortunately, they concentrated not only on the intended areas but also on my lung. My lung was clearly not an intended area of focus. As a result, the bottom line was that I would need to go have saline removed from my left side after all.

Cue the whistling noise of me sliding from space eighty-seven down to the bottom row.

My nice little treatment calendar was now null and void. All previous treatment plans were officially on hold. It was time to make calls and appointments to rectify the problem. I couldn't help but feel as though I was getting ready to plummet down the board. As for my week of events scheduled around appointment times? Moot. My first week of XRT done and under my belt by Friday? A distant memory.

I tried to convince myself that maybe it wasn't that bad, maybe the ray was only a tiny bit off and they'd just need to get rid of a mere 30 to 50 cc.

"How much do you need to remove?" I asked. He wasn't sure. He said that he would call my plastic surgeon in Boston and work with his partner and between the three of them, they would figure out how much to drain. He said I'd need to set up an appointment down there to have the saline taken out. After that was done, I needed to call him back so his staff could set me up with a new appointment, and, essentially, we'd start back at the beginning.

I headed out with my mind ablaze with a million thoughts, and he stopped me. He said, "We didn't want to call to tell you this. I wanted to tell you in person." I appreciated that. "It's just a little setback. Really, it's not a big deal." True, it wasn't, to him.

For me, every chute in this cancer journey started off as a big deal. It was always another readjustment that I had to make and accept, because there was nothing I could do about it. It was death by a thousand paper cuts. Each individual one hurt, stung, and burned. But, come on, it was just a paper cut! The burning would subside. It may or may not bleed or leave a scar. But each one sucked. And it would take a TON of paper cuts to kill me, so I knew I'd be in for the long haul. It was exhausting keeping my Zen, my happy place, my center intact when other people kept interfering. Logically, I knew that people weren't really interfering, they were helping. I knew that my radiology/oncology doctor was trying to spare me the heartache of having to go through an expander reduction (and everything that it would entail), and he tried to the best of his ability to avoid it. He could have burst my bubble from day one by telling me I had no choice. On my behalf, he tried to see if things would work as they were. As it turned out, it wasn't meant to be, and that was not *his* fault. But I did get my hopes up.

Now, not only would I have to make a new plan, I'd have to wait, get the new information, and THEN make a new plan. This may not have been a big deal and probably was a small glitch in the scheme of *his* piece of my treatment, but in the overall picture of the past five months, this was yet another pain-in-the-ass setback in a game with a set of rules that didn't seem to play out in my favor.

As I was getting into my car to head home, I tried to put my finger on at least ONE of the things whirling in my head so I could start to formulate a plan. First, I wanted to punch something, scream, cry, or maybe hold my breath until I passed out.

My solution was to go home and get on my elliptical trainer and run. This would allow endorphins, nature's little Xanax, to release the frustration and even me out. And I won't lie to you – Plan B *was* Xanax. As much as I wanted a glass of wine, if I gave in and had a drink every time I got stressed out, I'd be adding liver failure to my list of problems. The nice part about Xanax as a backup drug was that it washed away the anxiety. A short twenty minutes after ingestion, I felt like "Radiation shmay-diation, who needs it anyway? Not me." It put me in a nice little world to sit in as the immediacy of a situation I had no control over passed over me.

The next issue was that I had finally bonded with the expanders that I'd now had for five months. They were like the face(s) only a mother could love. After I had to have saline taken out, not only would I have expanders, I'd have *lopsided* expanders. Not that I had reason to believe that I'd be prancing around in a bathing suit all summer, but thinking ahead, I worried about the general ability to stay cool and comfortable in tank tops or summer sundresses. I feared it would become a logistical nightmare to try to hide the obvious asymmetry. The thought of granny bras and prosthetics made me angry and resentful. Not that a woman at any age deserves this, but I was too young for this crap.

The logical side of me knew that we *were* in the year 2012. My Aunt Leslie fits women with bras and breast prostheses in New Jersey. She said there were plenty of options available, and there were many modern, light, and fashionable prosthetic options for me. After all, it wasn't as if I'd have to chisel a rock down and place it in a pouch sewn under the chest of my wooly mammoth fur dress. But adding ONE more thing to my already altered body was overwhelming.

As I verbalized this frustration to Frieda, she said to me, "It's like you are running this marathon, and at the twenty-mile mark, someone stops you and says, 'Hey, I need your sneakers now.' So you give them your sneakers, and just as you're trying to figure out how to finish the race without sneakers, they stop you again and say, 'Oh, yeah, will you carry this knapsack, too?'" What next? Was it going to snow? It took all I had to run the race in the first place. Now, my resources were being stripped, and I was being asked to do more, with less.

The last issue was the timing of it all. How long would it be before I could get the appointment in Boston, then get back to treatment? Would it be put off for a week? Two? The longer the treatment was put off, the longer before I could heal and be ready for my final surgery, after which I could just get this all behind me.

Choices, choices. Which issue did I deal with first? After my appointment, I headed to my parents' house, where I was able to talk things through with my sister, mom, dad, and (Bonus!) Gee (my grandmother). I felt a bit better once I was able to talk to everyone. I went home to call to arrange the earliest appointment I could get in Boston, then get on my elliptical.

As soon as I got home, I found the number and placed a call to the scheduler of plastic surgery. When she answered and heard it was me, she said, "I was just going to call you." We briefly exchanged pleasantries, and then we got down to brass tacks.

She said, "Looks as if we need to schedule you to remove 110 cc from your contralateral expander."

I said, "No way."

She said, "No kidding."

Only I was saying "no way" not to be witty or funny, but more in an "Are you shitting me?" kind of way. "OK," I said, "Let's do this." She was able to get me in on Thursday, which meant I only had to wait until the day after next.

That conversation fired me up for a run on the elliptical. Every time my mind went to postponement, lopsidedness, prosthetics, or scheduling, I found myself taking it out on the machine. I was in a good place, with my eyes closed and my iPod cranked. Sixty-one minutes, four and three-quarter miles, and eighty-five crunches on the ab lounger later, I was feeling marginally better. At the very least, I no longer wanted to punch something.

While I was working out, Brian arrived home from work. I had yet to share with him not only the news of the earlier day's events but also of the more recent findings of how *much* I was going to have to have removed from my expander. We found a quiet spot, where the kids wouldn't be able to hear me if I had to cry. I verbalized all of my frustrations, my wtfs, my heartache, and my woes. Even after all of that exercising, I still ended up crying. Yet again, Brian listened and asked me how I was going to work through it. I said I was going to journal and write. His response was, "All beautiful things come from a place of suffering." *Did he mean my writing or me? That question I deem rhetorical.*

However, I was on edge the next few days. The waiting and in-between time weighed on me. I went from having a solid plan to floating in limbo. *What would I look like? Would I be able to or need to be fitted for a prosthesis? Would it be versatile? How much would that cost? How long would I be like that before I could be evened out? Would the asymmetry be obvious? Would it look ridiculous? Where was the good in this? There's always good hidden somewhere, right? What am I supposed to be learning here?* I just had to search.

Brian had taken Wednesday off in order to go with me to what was supposed to be my first day of radiation. Now, it was just a bonus day off. So, we decided to take a series of photos, not only to "document" this phase but to add a little more personality into it.

Somewhere out there, there is a woman about to embark on this journey, who, like me when I started all of this, doesn't know what expanders look like. Fishing through the internet can be scary. The internet is a blessing and a curse because it pulls up not only the helpful and positive, but also the negative and scary. Before surgery, I did a Google search, trying to find out what expanders might look like. Yikes. I wish I had known someone who had had them and could tell me that they weren't that bad.

Somewhere out there, there's a parent, spouse, sibling, or child of someone going through this process, someone who might be curious about what expanders look like and needs some reassurance. Maybe, there's someone who is bald, with no facial hair, or sprouting peach fuzz, someone who has lopsided expanders and needs to see that she's not alone. Maybe there are people out there who simply appreciate real, raw, artful footage of cancer and what it can do to you. I recently saw a black-and-white picture of a woman with two scars where her breasts used to be and a tattoo on her chest. I couldn't look away. It was beautiful, terrifying, and inspirational all at the same time. Maybe I could be that person for someone else like she was for me. Brian and I decided to shoot a series of photos with that in mind.

Although this seemed like a good idea to me, I wondered how my kids would react. What would they say if they saw pictures of their mother exposing her chest? I would think it would be a bit awkward, to say the least. So, I would have to tell them that I wanted to help others. I wanted to make a difference. If seeing and understanding the reality of what cancer does to a woman helped even one person without scaring her, and if these pictures moved people, we'd have done our job.

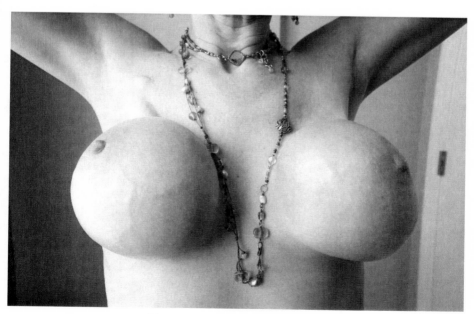

I know. It leaves you speechless . . .

I compared it to when I was breastfeeding. Although I was very discreet, if I needed to breastfeed in public and a random nipple went flopping out of my infant's mouth in a feeding frenzy, well, so be it. My breasts weren't sexual or provocative. They were utilitarian and just means to a functional end – to feed my infant. Period. If such a situation had been photographed, perhaps the raw beauty of a mother bonding with her infant could be captured. Just because a breast is in a photograph does not always mean it is sexual.

We took around three hundred photos of all kinds that Wednesday. In some, my expanders were exposed; others were just of me and my bald state. If beauty could be seen in the person underneath the bald head and irregular breast, then my job was done. So was Brian's. We hoped that somehow, they would touch people. I knew at the end of the day, I had found the good in this photo "chute." It forced us to take an opportunity to document this phase of my journey, which I would not have normally done.

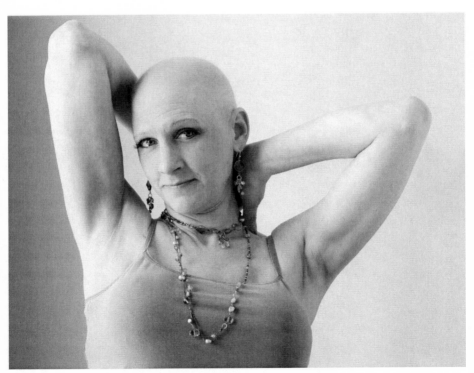

Embracing body image with a photo shoot, bald with expanders

Friday's trip to Boston couldn't come soon enough. I started my day trying to work to the best of my ability, but I couldn't get my head around my job. I answered emails and made phone calls and worked on a project or two, but then I ended up taking a Xanax because of an anxiety I just couldn't shake.

I met Frieda at the Park and Ride, and we drove to Boston together. We talked, she made me laugh, and she calmed me down with her very funny yet matter-of-fact demeanor. I got to see the nurse practitioner, whom I loved. In spite of the wig, she immediately recognized me and said, "Wow, it's been a while since I've seen you." It was nice to be remembered. She brought us in to the exam room and had two scripts already printed out for my prosthesis and mastectomy bra. (Apparently, you need a prescription for them!) She said that their scheduler had told her that I was interested in them, and so the ARNP had them ready for me, regardless of whether I would use them. She excused herself, I changed into the gown, and then returned.

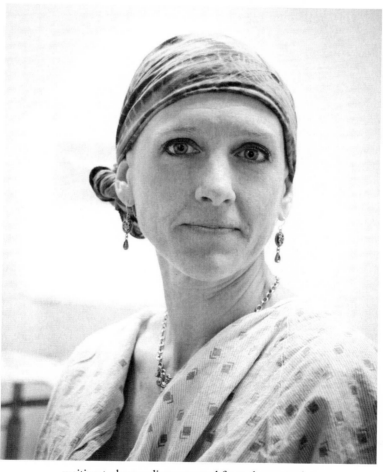

waiting to have saline removed from the expander

Before she started, I asked her what the total volume was in each expander. She had to look it up on the computer. While she did, I talked to her about the plastic surgeons she worked with. I let her know I was having a hard time warming up to mine, and I asked what type of experience she had with that surgeon. I also asked if there was one surgeon who did more post-mastectomy implant surgeries than the others. She was professional and very straight with me. I was not looking to have her "dish" about my surgeon. I did believe that she has exceptional surgical talent, or she wouldn't be working at a tertiary hospital. I wasn't looking to speak ill of her, either.

I had to keep reminding myself, as did the ARNP (and many others as well) that it is OK to get a second opinion. It is the smart thing to do. You have to feel good about the person performing your surgery. I believe that an outcome can rely partly on your attitude about the surgery, and if you are not on board with your surgeon, that doesn't lend well to overall healing. She gave me two business cards of other doctors she felt had exceptional bedside manners in addition to being great surgeons, and she said if I wanted to do a little research and meet with either of them, to let her know. She said that sometimes providing a little background to the surgeon is helpful to them.

That personal connection made it much easier to have the saline removed. She aspirated the 110 cc and told me that as soon as I was done with radiation, I could come right back and they would put it back in! *Holy super symmetrical summer, Batman! That was great news!* I glanced at my newly shaped breast, and it actually looked more like a breast than a shiny, skin-colored rock. It had a little give and felt a little more like a real breast, too. It was a little weird, don't get me wrong, but it was almost like my left breast was saying, "Ahhhh, *thank you* for the break." I left with my questions answered, I had leads, and I was getting my mojo back, regardless of the reality that I now had a notably smaller, squishier left boob.

I had the foresight to call ahead to the boutique at the hospital and make an appointment to be fitted for a prosthesis. The timing was perfect. As we left the appointment with the ARNP, I had just enough time to get to the boutique in the next building for my 3:45 appointment. In the "Images Boutique," there were wigs, bras, prostheses, creams, clothes, and breast cancer swag galore. There, I met with a lady, who appeared to be all hopped up on the bean (and perhaps needed to try some decaf). She was very friendly and brought us in the back room and proceeded to talk a mile a minute. (I mentioned to Brian that she didn't stop talking from the minute we saw her, and his fun-loving response was, "Huh, I wonder what that's like." I know. I do the same thing. He got me there.) She talked about the styles of bras, the skin's reaction to radiation immediately after treatment and further down the road, the swelling, the need for a bra, creams and lotions, and handy little pieces of advice like, use corn starch – not talc powder – and don't combine lotion and corn starch or you'll end up with a paste, put lotion on a baby washcloth and put it in the refrigerator so it would be cool and soothe my skin after treatment, and and and . . . .

Thankfully, the first bra/prosthetic I tried on was a winner, and although she had a plethora (and then some) of information to share, my head was hurting from the speed in which it was being delivered. I handed her my script, and no money needed to exchange hands. I asked if I could get another later on if need be. She said yes, but I may want to wait . . . and started her speed talking again. I don't recall why she suggested I wait, but I knew that with all of her talking that I was ready to go. (In retrospect, I don't know why I didn't get two. I mean, what woman can live on one bra and one bra alone?)

I wore my new bra and "prosthesis" out of the store looking inconspicuous but feeling I had a secret. It was far from a rock in a pouch under my wooly mammoth fur dress; it was good. Feeling normal, I had a very relaxing ride home.

Friday, I took my mapping mulligan. I went in unsure of what exactly I was going in for. The doctor told me it would be a re-mapping, and we'd be re-doing everything but the tattoos, only this time things would go faster because it was essentially a repeat of what we did before. In addition, it was not going to take the full week to work the 3-D image with the physicist. This was good news, because I should be able to do the sim verification sooner and therefore start radiation sooner.

The receptionist checked me in, and after changing into a johnny, I went back to the same room as before, where the radiology technician rescanned me. This time I asked questions. What exactly was she doing? And why? She took the time to take a piece of paper to show me the laser beams and how she was trying to line them up for the scan. I felt much more comfortable and informed. After all was done, she disappeared to create a schedule for me. Her first proposition reflected that I wasn't going to have the sim verification until the following Thursday, and because they didn't start actual radiation on a Friday (because it would mean needing to have two days off right away), I wouldn't start until the fifth of the following month! She read my face and said, "Is that not good for you?" I told her I was told that this time, I wasn't supposed to have to wait as long for the verification. I found out that she had only done it that way to try to accommodate the fact that I had requested a time around 2:30. I told her it was more important to make a few concessions to scheduling if I could get things started earlier. She came back with a revised schedule, and I now had verification on Tuesday and would start Wednesday. The schedule time varied the first few weeks, but I would eventually get onto a regular schedule. For now, I was glad I was ON a schedule at all. My ducks were back in a row.

So there I was, playing a competitive yet methodical game with my cancer recovery. I encountered a few little ladders that boosted me ahead, only to find as I hit a rhythm that a chute would set me back. I wasn't lucky enough to hit the golden staircase that would give me a fast track to the final row on the chutes and ladders board of life, but that was OK. In retrospect, I needed to be sent back down the chute so that I could spend time with the nurse practitioner, who helped put my surgeon choice worries at ease, as well as take photographs with Brian that solidified my desire to have something formal published. I reached out to an old friend, Melissa, who is in the "editing business." She helped me brainstorm and navigate through getting started and offered to help me along the way. I also spoke to a publishing company. I wanted to make a difference, and now I would. I know now, in retrospect, that I was sent down the "big chute" because all beautiful things do come from suffering and hard work.

CHAPTER TWENTY-TWO

Cowhorn Cancer

Saturday, March 17, 2012

For Shannon and Tom

YEARS AGO, WHEN the kids were young (Samantha, Abbie, and Donald were around twelve, nine, and six, respectively), we would look forward to weekend nights, where we could venture over to our good friends' and neighbors' house for "Casino Night." They had a mini-roulette wheel, Blackjack, "Texas Hold 'Em," and Tom, the best bartender in town. Although their children were younger than ours, the atmosphere was always kid friendly, with things for Sam, Abbie, and Don to do – from movies to games to the occasional participation in the adult gambling games. Who isn't fascinated by a roulette wheel?

On one particular visit, Donald decided he wanted to play a card game, too. Because teaching him the particulars of the button, the flop, the turn, and the river seemed beyond our abilities, Tom obliged Donald to a card game of Donald's choice.

A red deck of cards with a black silhouette of a bull was handed to Don. He dealt the cards and explained the rules of the game in six-year-old fashion. From the explanation, it appeared that it was a "learn as you go" sort of game, so, intrigued and entertained by the prospects of this nebulous game, Tom ran with it. The two of them competitively played the first hand as Tom got his sea legs. But it was over before it started . . . Don crushed him in the first round. I think the score was around twenty to nothing. But Donald's intense determination to explain the game, combined with Tom's fun-loving, fatherly nature, quickly led to a second hand. As the cards were being dealt, Tom asked, "Donald, what exactly is the name of this game?" Don sat and thought about it for a second. He and Tom simultaneously caught a glance of the bull on the back of the cards, and Don replied, "Cowhorn." Tom nodded, and with an "I should have known" look on his face, said, "Ah-haaaa! Very clever."

The second hand went a bit better for Tom. He had a general handle on the rules, and, sympathetic to the fragility of his pre-pubescent opponent, he double-checked to confirm with Don that he'd earned a legit point before he allowed himself to officially take it. Soon, it was neck and neck . . . the excitement mounted . . . and . . . just as the score was a point or two from being even . . . BAM! Don changed the rules. Suddenly, what had applied in the previous hand was not only null and void but 180 degrees different. It didn't take long to realize that there was no way to win . . . the name of the game was to hang on to as much dignity as possible until the game was over. Thankfully, Donald's attention span was short and the game didn't last long. Tom shook his hand and said, "Good game. Thank you for playing." Don walked away pleased as punch, and Tom swiped his forehead and said, "Thank GOD that's over!"

Although Cowhorn may never have its own table in Vegas, the term has been fondly incorporated into our lives now whenever we're dealing with something that changes just when we think we know what we're doing. Luckily, saying the mere word "Cowhorn" still makes me laugh at the memory and can ease the intensity of a stressful moment.

Cancer treatment lives in the Cowhorn bucket. From the treatment side effects to the appointments that depend on the outcome of another to the constant readjusting the line of normal, it's all a big bucket of Cowhorn. As I said, just when you think you know the rules, they change. And you adapt to each and every phase you have to go through as you sit on the edge of your seat, waiting for the rules to change again.

At the beginning, the Cowhorn intensity was much higher. I think that with fatigue and healing, combined with chemotherapy drugs, one's system is the most compromised, and it is easy to feel the slightest degree of any little change. At this point in my recovery, although the frustrations of change came in waves, they weren't twenty-foot waves that could swallow a person whole; they were more the five-foot waves that you can try to ride but often still knock you over.

I started radiation therapy (XRT) as part of "Phase Three" of treatment. (To recap: I had the original mastectomy, then chemotherapy, and was now doing the radiation. Last would be the final surgery.) I was told that the side effects of the radiation therapy would be primarily "sunburn" and fatigue. Great. I'd been told by friends that the area being radiated is very uniform. It is mapped out on the body roughly in the form of a rectangle, perhaps a rhomboid, or maybe even a parallelogram that reddens like a sunburn on the breast. It happens gradually, and, according to the radiation technicians, it would start to show about the second to third week. They suggested a few different creams and lotions to help with the burn. The chatty lady in Boston had suggested that when the burn started to feel uncomfortable, I should keep baby washcloths coated with lotion in the fridge and apply them after treatment for a cool, soothing option. I was also told that it may be helpful to stop wearing a bra and trade it for a silky camisole, because the rubbing of the sides can be very uncomfortable. Yeah, right. A silky camisole.

I appreciated these options, honestly I did. I'm sure they help many women. But if I didn't wear a bra, I might as well have had someone shine a spotlight on my chest and hold a neon sign above my head that said, "Look at how lopsided she is!" The idea of a silk camisole was about as realistic as me becoming a "Solid Gold" dancer. It was hard enough to "even the girls out" when I was wearing a bra, never mind when I wasn't.

I must admit, though, that the lopsidedness didn't bother me as much as I thought it would. At this point, it was like accepting the fact that my nipples pointed in different directions – it was what it was. And at least I still had nipples.

For those who have not undergone chemo, the fatigue from radiation starts at about three weeks after the first treatment. But for those who have had chemo, it starts earlier. How much? I'm not really sure. The answer is always, "It's different for each individual." But in my case, I was utterly exhausted after having treatments for only a week and a half.

I was told that one thing known to help fatigue is regular exercise. That's easy enough, right? It isn't like giving up chocolate. I wanted to be strong and healthy and do whatever I could to avoid the fatigue. As I've mentioned before, fatigue isn't just being tired. It isn't necessarily treated by taking a quick nap or sleeping in. It can be like a ball and chain attached to each of your legs as you drag them around behind you. Personally speaking, fatigue affected my motivation, my abilities, my productivity, and my emotions. It made the difference between a well thought-out and balanced meal and ordering pizza, achieving all goals of the day or just one or two, and laughing off a little well-intended, fun-loving banter or landing in a bucket of tears. If the fatigue I'd experienced to this point was any indication of what I could avoid going forward, exercise sounded like a great idea.

It was the season of Lent. A season to reflect and think about how to be a better person and be more pleasing to God. I had "given up" things in the past. For example, I gave up wine one year and swearing another. Shamefully, the swearing was the harder of the two. (Who knew I had such a potty mouth!) But Lent isn't always about giving something up; it is about reflecting on how to be a better Christian, so sometimes, it is more about what you *should* do than what you *shouldn't*. Either way, I "gave up" *not* exercising for Lent. To be healthier and serve my purpose as a mother, friend, daughter, co-worker, and Christian, I would exercise. God gave me strength to get through this. I would do my part.

Very lucky for me, I learned that as a patient at the cancer center, I'd be given three months *free* at the hospital-owned gym a few miles up the street. There is an actual program offered called the "Cancer Recovery" program. Melanie, the kind-spirited woman there who ran the program, offered classes three times a week that incorporated weight training, stretching, and a cardio workout. The down side was that it was from 12:30 to 1:30 pm on Mondays, Wednesdays, and Fridays. Exercise was yet another thing to add into my already filled days. My radiation schedule didn't regulate to a "normal" time until the following week, and until then, the Cancer Recovery program fell right in the middle of my workday. I decided that I would like a little bit more of a challenge than what the basic program offered.

I was also driven by the fact that I would be having reconstructive surgery in the late summer or early fall, and I didn't want my new breasts to be the best part of me. It would stink if my body were equivalent to a woman all dressed up in an elegant evening gown but wearing Timberland boots on her feet for shoes, or a rusted-out car with a shiny new chrome bumper. (Visuals for both the male and females out there . . . you're welcome.) I talked to Melanie, and she was happy to work out an individual plan to meet my personal goals, due to my scheduling difficulties and exercise level. She walked me through all of the various machines and options for what I was looking to achieve, yet was sensitive to the fact that I still had a port, which could cause me problems. She encouraged me to stick with certain machines until that was removed. Best of all, she TOTALLY buttered me up by saying that she wasn't used to working with an "athlete!" My kids are athletes, but I haven't been called that for a *long* time! I don't think she knew how that simple description motivated me. We came up with a challenging workout, and my goal was to go to the gym three times a week.

The thing was, I was now at the cancer center five days a week for treatment. My offices for work were only a few miles up the street from the gym, and I passed by them every day to go to radiation. To NOT go in and do at least a little something seemed wrong. The sign at the gym out by the road that lit up with new messages and specials each week and month might as well read, "Really, Tracy? You are going to pass right by and not stop in?" The hardest part about exercising is committing to doing it and getting there. Once you're there, even if you have a crappy workout, it was a workout. And you are left thinking, "Huh, that was crappy; I'll do better next time."

The week before was a busy week. It was jam packed with work deadlines and expectations (albeit many of them self-inflicted) and my first full week of radiation. Unfortunately, the open time slots so far had been smack in the middle of the day *around* lunchtime . . . but not quite. I'm not really a morning person, so trying to get my momentum going was a daily challenge, even on my best days.

Inevitably, just as I would start to feel awake and find my stride, my phone alarm would go off to tell me it was time to leave for treatment. I needed about thirty minutes to get there and park, then fifteen minutes to register and get changed. The actual treatment itself lasted less than fifteen minutes. Then I would change back to work clothes again and head back to the office.

Picking up where I left off was a challenge, too. I'd return to my desk, sit down, and stare at the computer screen. *Now, where was I again? I'm not really sure, but I probably shouldn't re-start anything before I eat my lunch; otherwise, I'll just get started and be distracted by hunger pains until I eat.* And of course, stopping to eat would break my stride. Again. There is a lot to be said about getting a momentum going and keeping it.

To add insult to injury, it was a busy emotional week with personal issues, concerns as a mother, worries as a partner, stresses as an employee, and all the bills were due. You know those weeks. I'm pretty sure that in my normal world, they generally fell on the week where I was premenstrual and had the patience of a pea – every last thing irritated me. (Due to my premature menopause, I think my moods cycled with the moon.) And so, why not . . . this seemed like a GREAT time to throw in a new routine, including packing for the gym (and remembering things like sneakers, socks, iPod, water bottle, and a regular bandana to cover my baby hair fuzz), daily workouts, radiation, smoothies for breakfast, and packing daily lunches. I wouldn't be tired by any of that, right? I felt as if I were giving up smoking, drinking, and a drug and chew habit while starting a new job and relationship and buying a house. OK, that might be slightly overstated, but it was one of those weeks where I was exhausted, and one of about a million things could have been the culprit. Because, it couldn't possibly already be the effects of the XRT, right? Something needed to give, but what was the right thing to give up?

My particular dilemma was that I had the whole "chicken and the egg" thing going. In order to battle fatigue, I needed to exercise. In order to exercise, I needed to find time in an already busy schedule and organize myself further and make adjustments so I could take advantage of this great, free opportunity. And that was exhausting. (As is, might I add, *exercising* when you're not used to it.) Maybe I wouldn't be tired if I just said, "Screw it," and left the whole exercise piece behind. Now was the time to get into a healthy habit, one that was good for me and would help me in the long term if I kept it up. But somebody please tell me, who the hell left ME in charge of moderating how much I should be doing? Clearly, I sucked at it. I had to make my own mistakes, evidently by doing too much and ending up in a puddle of tears before I could reflect and say, "Well, I guess I was trying to do too much this week. Let's try again next week."

I thought I knew what was best for me, but my busy person personality didn't allow me to do just a little; it didn't feel right to have down time, or "me" time or "free" time. It felt comfortable only when I was on the go from when I woke until it was time for bed. Old habits are hard to break, right? When I thought about it,

I wasn't really surprised to realize that I was (yet again) experiencing impatience with the healing and treatment process. I came out of the ups and downs of the chemo schedule with renewed strength and energy, so I thought I should give it a shot to try to "beat" the next phase and not let it get me down. Therefore, I found myself ignoring the signs of being tired and needing to slow down a bit.

It got a bit better. I got into a groove and gave myself permission to relax and not exercise on Wednesdays. It was a great balance. I felt energized when I left the gym; I'd just treated myself to something healthy and good for me. And it allowed me to feel tired from something normal and healthy rather than something *cancer*-related, like radiation treatments. I gained some power from that – instead of feeling like a victim of radiation, I felt like a triumphant conqueror of a healthy habit. So, when I got home, if I was tired, it felt OK to relax or even take a power nap, because I was being good to myself with exercise.

With Cowhorn cancer treatment, you think you know the rules and what to expect, but they change with the day. Anticipating a straightforward week was simply a set-up for a swift kick in the Cowhorn . . . with disappointing results. The key to Cowhorn, in any event, is riding with the unpredictable flow and anticipating that nothing is written in stone. The play is fluid, and there is a lesson to be learned, however small, with every hand. I conclude that if you can play the hand through and laugh in the end, you've really won the game.

CHAPTER TWENTY THREE

The Final Countdown

Sunday, April 1, 2012

THE LAST FEW weeks brought a new set of discoveries – physical, mental, and social.

On the up side, I could now officially say I had hair. It was shorter than a crew cut, and the color was still unidentifiable, but it was there, even if it did look as if I had a serious case of hat head without wearing the hat. My eyebrows and hair matched, and once my eyelashes started growing, they grew quickly. I no longer had to search for little stubs to brush mascara over or wear false eyelashes.

And once the hair "switch" was turned on, it sure made up for lost time. Not only had my leg and underarm hair returned, but I discovered fine "baby hair" not only on my head but on the edges of my cheeks and jaw line and down the sides and back of my neck. (Sexy!) Although it was soft, fine, bleach-blonde hair, when it caught the sunlight just right, I looked like a blonde, female Grizzly Adams. (Not really the look I was hoping for.) On a positive note, I was fortunate that it was blonde, because if it were dark, I'd need to join the circus. I can't believe I am saying this, but I actually hoped it would fall out – or at least that it would thin – as fine baby hair does. I didn't know if it was all that noticeable to others as it was to me, but geez. It seemed to be all or nothing these days.

I was transiently brave with the hair. I wanted to walk out of the house one day and just rock the über short hair look. But instead, I had brave moments where I would do things like answer the door when the UPS man delivered a package or go to the cardio room at the gym with nothing on my head. I now often took off my wig or headscarf on my drive home from work. However, one time, I "got brave" by accident. I was working around the house (where I generally didn't wear anything on my head) and had to make a quick trip to the grocery store. I was in my car at the end of the street, about to turn onto the main road, before I realized, "Hey, wait! I don't have anything on my head!" Abbie was with me and said, "Just go like this; you look beautiful." So I did.

I know I am harder on myself than others are. I tried to keep a low profile, but Abbie saw people we knew and made it a point to say, "Hey Mom, there is Mrs. F!" and before I knew it, we'd gotten her attention from three aisles over. The next thing I knew, I was checking out and having a conversation with Mrs. F over all of the cashiers and baggers as she made her way out of the store. It ended up being a positive experience, because she said she had seen me from a ways away and wondered who the woman was with the chic short haircut. I believe she meant it, but even if she was being nice, I didn't really care. It was just what I needed, and she made my evening.

I had my port removed on March 23. It was an office procedure, which was a bit daunting, because it was put IN in the hospital under general anesthesia. I was numbed up locally, and I was amazed to feel how many adhesions had formed to the metal port itself where it had been sewn in. I say, "feel," because most of the time during the procedure, I could feel the surgeon scraping the adhesions off the port to free it before he could take it out. (I didn't look at it but talked to him through the whole thing . . . WITH Xanax on board, just in case.) It sounds gross. But it wasn't bad. There was one time when I realized the local anesthetic wasn't covering all of the area, but as soon as I said I felt it, he numbed that area with another injection, and within seconds, the pain went away. I got to see what the torture device looked like once it was out. I immediately felt better. The site burned like a fresh incision for a few days, but nothing that didn't abate with regular Tylenol. Once it was gone, I was able to regain better range of motion in my right arm. It served its purpose, and I am very glad I had it for the chemo. But I was equally as glad when it was removed.

I still received daily radiation treatment. Even though it was initially a disruption to my daily schedule, dare I say that it had actually become enjoyable? Although the actual procedure was not painful and didn't induce anything unpleasant like nausea or a metallic taste, the worst of it was that nine out of ten times, my arms fell asleep above my head. OK, I know what you're thinking. "Oh, the horror of pins and needles in your arms, Tracy. That must be awful." It wasn't. I appreciated that the procedure itself was a piece of cake, and (as I've mentioned earlier), other than my arms falling asleep, the fatigue, sunburn, and disruption to the day were the hardest parts of this piece. I have to say, it was the *staff* who made the leg of this journey so much more palatable.

The front desk receptionist came to know me and always welcomed me by name and with a smile before I could even make my way to her desk. The registration women were very social, good at making upbeat small talk and remembering details of my life. I felt as if they knew me; they were always happy to see me, no matter who checked me in and sent me down the hall. Their light and cheerful conversations make me feel like a healthy person, not a patient, and I liked it when they commented on an outfit or my energy level, which was usually pretty good by that time.

In the waiting room, I made new friends and got to know the faces and names of the other women who were dressed identical to me from the waist up. We chatted, caught up, shared stories, talked about treatments, and counted down the days with each other. One woman informed me that the weird change I was experiencing with my fingernails was from chemo, and lo and behold, hers looked just like mine! Another finally got her prosthetic "boob" and was none too shy about sharing that tidbit with contagious enthusiasm with anyone in the waiting area! She showed off her stylish "boob bag" where she put it when she changed into her gown for treatment. Another woman who'd just begun treatment asked me questions about the process, as well as the check-in and dependability of the staff running on time. It just so happened that on her second day, a simple light bulb *in* the machine blew out, and the staff had to call in a special person to take apart the machine to change it. This resulted in abnormal delay of fifteen minutes. Almost every time I'd been there, I was called in early.

Another very thin woman who could not sit down normally due to pain waited patiently for the one section of extra wide, side-by-side seating to free up so that she could stretch out and sort of lie down on her side. She never asked anyone to move; she simply stood, gently rocking back and forth, and good-naturedly waited until the seat became available. I watched her do this on her second-to-last day without realizing why she did it. When the previous occupant headed for treatment and the seat was freed, I patted the newly vacated extra-wide seat next to me and said, "Come on over and sit down now." It was then that we struck up a conversation and I found that it was too painful for her to sit normally. You get a feel early on as to how much people want to share, if anything. I don't know what kind of cancer she had, but learned she was nearing the finish line the next day. I asked if she had more treatment, and she said she didn't know yet. I realized how lucky I was that at least I knew my course.

In the waiting room, a number of us post-chemo recipients discussed hair details: the fascination of re-growth, the color, the texture, the products to use, and the feeling of going out into public with a hairstyle that wasn't quite chemo head but hadn't reached "trés chic" level, either. In my case, as I mentioned earlier, it was more of a non-style of its own that lay flat in whatever direction it wanted. (Unless of course, you count that one totally white rogue hair that was twice as long as the rest and stood straight out above my ear. Chic factor: zero!) I wish I could say that I was rocking it like Halle Berry did when her hair was short short . . . but not so much.

In the waiting room, we could openly share our situations and experiences. It was a great group of women, and we had our own private support group.

The radiation/oncology nurses checked in with me at least once before my visit with the doctor, but many times, they visited more often. One was a particular help and gave me a lot of extra support. She too was a breast cancer survivor. She got it. She was in the same age range as me and helped me with very important (and often taboo) things like sexuality. She understood the post-chemo-induced menopause and how it was quick and intense and added to my already frustrated state of mind with obvious body alterations. She actually followed up with me periodically. She gave me a couple of books and pamphlets that were very helpful. When I asked, she talked about her own personal experiences and provided helpful resources. I have said before that I met a number of people I would have chosen as a friend had I met them in my neighborhood or at a cookout. She was one of them.

Lastly, the radiation technicians were awesome. Even a twenty-minute encounter, five days a week, can result in some level of friendship. For the first day of spring, there were signs posted all around for everyone to wear their brightest colors. One of the techs wore a multi-neon colored feather boa! It was great and such a fun talking point. I got to know these women as well. We talked about everything from food to workouts to our kids to general funny stories. They asked about my day and seemed genuinely interested in the answer. They were always smiling, or so it seemed. They made the trip social (which was a plus for me), and although they talked over me as they confirmed my positioning and left the room three different times, they engaged me as much as possible. It was more personal attention than I got in a normal day at work. So, I guess I can say, actual treatment aside, the overall "disruption" to my daily schedule balanced out with wonderful people to socialize with and was, in fact, very much worth it.

I saw my radiation oncologist once a week. He was always encouraging, smiling, asking me if anything unexpected had happened. In that aspect, I was very prepared. He reported his opinion of the condition of my skin, and, contrary to my own belief, he said it not only looked great, but better than expected. You know you have an unusual set of circumstances when "great and better than expected" is an angry shade of purple instead of normal skin color. From under my right armpit to the middle of my ribs, over across my whole right breast, I had discoloration. They prepared me for sunburn. This was a sunburn I had never encountered . . . and I am from the teenage sit-in-the-sun-slathered-with-baby-oil era. Granted, I quickly became all about the SPF 30-45, but even back then, I don't recall a burn this bad. Where the underarm of a tank top or a bra would go was a deep, dark, purple raw area. And painful. I-can't-put-my-arm-down-without-pain painful . . . the equivalent to road rash under my arm.

I scoffed when the radiation therapist told me a couple of weeks previously to entertain the use of a silk camisole instead of a bra. NOW I was pickin' up what she was puttin' down! Suddenly, the "being lopsided" concern took a backseat to any form of comfort. I had to tap into creative dressing strategies. Wearing any type of bra, even a tank top with a "shelf bra," was painful because it rubbed on the raw part. That made exercise a challenge, because the support tops rubbed on the sore areas, too. Even though structurally, I really didn't need one, somehow it felt wrong not to wear *something*.

I had a plethora of creams, gels, and lotions to put on the sore areas. However, what brought me the most comfort was natural, homegrown aloe vera. I asked a friend who has a number of plants for a few leaves. She generously gave me a plastic container with about seven large ones. I put them in the fridge. When I was hurting, I cut off a four-to-five inch piece, sliced off the prickly edge, sliced the leaf lengthwise, and put it, goopy inner-side of the leaf down, directly on my skin. I actually secured them inside my bra so it kept the aloe there. Although it felt like heaven, I walked around wanting to tell a secret no one knew. (*Pssst . . . does anything about me seem strange to you? Because I have a PLANT hidden in my shirt! How terribly random! But shhh . . . don't tell anyone!*)

Steve Martin had a stand-up routine that I loved as a teen. When someone asked him once how he could be so f***ing funny, he said that he put a piece of bologna in his shoes, so he FELT funny. Aloe in the bra yielded a similar feeling. I knew the aloe secret was safe unless I got into an accident on my way home. Picture the scenario: the EMTs find me in the car, alive and breathing of course (I couldn't die in a car wreck after all of this, for Pete's sake). They'd strategically place their stethoscopes to listen to my breath sounds in all quadrants of my lung, then notice my aloe vera lump and say, "what the . . . hey, get a load of this. I think this woman hit an aloe tree. She's got a lump of aloe stuck to her side."

Although my skin was purple and raw, I believed the aloe juice helped heal it. (I'm not sure of the proper term . . . is it juice or nectar?) I had an area on my collarbone on the right side where they focused on the lymph nodes, as well as an area on my back where the radiation beams actually went *through* me and exited my back. It was red and looked as if I'd missed a spot when applying sunscreen. My clavicle was red and blistering, and the breast, well, it had looked better. The skin was red and looked like a rash. All over. The up side was that because my nerves were cut, I had decreased sensation on my breast. And I didn't lose my breath from the shock of applying cold aloe straight out of the fridge. It was also a good reminder that if I were ever to drop a scalding hot cup of coffee on my chest, I'd need to pay attention because I wouldn't feel it, and it could badly burn me and I wouldn't even know it. I was told that one to two weeks after treatment, it would still continue to get worse before it got better. It looked as if I'd have a few creative clothing weeks ahead of me.

For nine months, I'd been thinking about my last day of treatment. I'd be freed from the clenches of cancer treatment and the crucial need to follow the plan through to the end in order to minimize and alleviate my chances of recurrence. Nine months ago, I was looked straight in the eye and told, "You have a BIG tumor; we need to get it out as quickly as we can and get started right away on treatment to prevent recurrence." I didn't take that lightly; it was the most serious assignment that I'd ever been issued. I committed to doing whatever it took and didn't look back.

So, I altered priorities, rearranged plans, and shuffled schedules. Make way for the new life! Admittedly, it wasn't that easy. As you may recall, I went down metaphorically kicking and screaming as I conceded to some of those tasks, thinking I really wouldn't have to alter that much to get to the other side. (Eye roll.) I kept in mind that "everything was temporary." I have found that you can do almost anything if you know there is light at the end of the tunnel and that you only have to endure the bad stuff for a finite amount of time.

The reality of my treatment coming to a close hit me one particular week. I met with my radiation oncologist for my weekly visit. He came in with his bright white smile and said, "Can you believe it? Seventeen down and eleven to go." Wow! Holy cow. Really? Then what? Then, I'm afraid, the new norm cast a strange and foreign shadow when the familiarity of active treatment slammed on its brakes and came to a violent and screeching halt. Not only did it come to a screeching halt, but I was also kicked to the curbside while my trusty ride sped off into the sunset in a cloud of dust to become nothing more than a distant memory. I didn't feel ready. I felt ill equipped.

For nine months, I felt secure and supported by the strict regimen of treatment. Every month, every week, every day, I scheduled my life and responsibilities around said treatment, because I took it seriously and wanted the best outcome; the most important thing was to get it and carry it out to the letter of the law. Appointments, academic activities, sports events, holidays, and workdays were all juggled around treatment. It was my life. It was serious shit.

Then, one day, it would end. Boom. My entire oncology team would give me the "all clear" and tell me I was good to go. Bub-bye. It was like driving a car at ninety miles per hour and hitting a wall. You're just suddenly . . . done? Monday would be a normal routine of lunch at 12:30, leave work at 1:45, check in at 2:15, radiation therapy at 2:30, exercise at 3:15, and get home around 5:00. On Tuesday, that schedule of the past six weeks would be a distant memory. Weird. Now, what?

When I was in the Navy, a high-ranking officer would occasionally visit our busy Medical-Surgical floor. When he or she arrived, the first person to notice was to stand at attention and respectfully yell, "Attention on Deck!" Upon hearing that command, everyone was to stop what they were doing and stand at attention. The high-ranking officer "released" us with a command of, "As you were," or "carry on." On a busy Med-Surg nursing floor, it meant everyone could return to tending patients. The world of a soldier paused momentarily as due respect and recognition were displayed to the "brass" (i.e., the high-ranking officer).

At the end of my treatment, I felt as though I were about to be given the "as you were" command from the universe, releasing me to "carry on" as though the last nine months were only a momentary lapse of time in my life. That I needed to proceed as if nothing happened. How did I do that?

Ideally, I think it would have been nice if they could have weaned me off treatment slowly. When you are prescribed certain steroids, you start off at full strength, then eventually wean from two pills a day, to one pill a day for a few days, then one pill every other day, then a half pill every other day, and THEN you're done. That would have been ideal to allay my anxieties around this sudden cessation of treatment. Because, for me, there were no further tests to be done to be SURE the cancer was all gone and all of the treatments had worked successfully. I just had to assume it worked and pick up my recently altered self and go home and live life on my own. Sure, they threw me a bone and reminded me of my follow-up appointment with my medical oncologist at the end of April, but other than that, I had to believe I really was all set unless something awful told me otherwise. All those reassuring daily, or at least weekly, trips to the hospital were now gone, and I was no longer going to do anything ACTIVE to fight this cancer, because, by this point, it was all gone. Or so everyone assumed.

All of those supportive, smiling faces with whom I laughed and engaged in daily conversation, and who made me feel so very cared for, would go on supporting others who had that "new cancer smell." I, on the other hand, would walk away with only a faint smell of "johnny" and sufficiently burnt flesh. When I was gone, my 2:30 slot would be filled with the next person in need of treatment. In my mind, I WAS the 2:30 person, but really, I was only a blink of an eye in the scheme of patients rolling through for their treatment. I felt like a first-time gladiator dressed in impractical heels and work attire who has been shoved out into the Coliseum, armed with a bottle of perfume and an electric razor, waiting for the doors on the opposite side of the pit to open.

Did I have what I needed to survive now? On the one hand, yes, I think I did. I mean, how hard could it be? All I had to do was put one foot in front of the other. But on the other hand, I was so comfortable with the surroundings of my constant medical regimen that I couldn't foresee the end . . . and now it was here and I wasn't prepared for this phase. It's a huge phase, because it's the rest of my life. It's life after cancer.

When you take a class, you spend hours of time learning your new subject. You perhaps listen, read, and absorb all there is to know about your subject. You prepare yourself for the final test, take said test, and then, if all goes well, you're able to apply what you've learned in your next real-life situation. At this point, I had six treatments left. My last day, my final test, was a little more than a week away – I should feel relief. I should feel like celebrating, right? I had wanted a celebration when I was done with my chemo, and I expected to feel the same way when I was done with radiation. But instead, I feel oddly unprepared for life after treatment. It was as if I had to take a test for a subject that I not only didn't study for, but I also didn't attend the classes, or get the text book, or even know that I enrolled in the class in the first place. I felt a sense of impending doom, and I hoped common sense would get me through.

I'd been reading *After Breast Cancer: A Common-Sense Guide to Life After Treatment* by Hester Hill Schnipper (New York: Bantam, 2006). I could relate to the feelings and worries carefully written there. But one thing especially resonated with me: "things will never be as they were before cancer." I mentioned before that cancer is a game changer. But somehow, through all of this, I always maintained that I just wanted my old body back – I wanted things to be as they were, and that is what I strived for. I liked both my body and my life. I realize now that I needed to change my thinking a little, because, really, life would never be the same as it was. I had to believe it would be better because I was now stronger.

Some of my friends, relatives, and acquaintances have had cancer and, had I not known, I never would have guessed because of how they carried on with their lives. Would I have that appearance? Was this an exclusive club whose members are the only ones who know how to pull this off gracefully? (If I'm let in, I hope that the secret club handshake includes the "baby bird" and a bootie shake because I love those two moves.) I want in. I have experienced the "it won't ever happen to me" scenario.

As positive of an attitude as I have, that damn seed of worry was planted, and even Jack Bauer can't unring that bell. Although I didn't plan to feed it with worry, it was there, and exactly how could I ignore it? With thoughts like, *Will I remain cancer free forever? Will it hit again next year, or in ten years, or twenty-five? Will my mother, sister, or children have to go through this?* looming in my head, I guess the only way to keep it at bay was to not give it undeserved attention. Don't worry about things that have not yet happened. Most of the time, that was doable. But there were random moments where it was utterly paralyzing.

Going into my last full week of radiation, I was like a squirrel frantically gathering nuts before the winter, trying to collect as much as I could to help me through the transition to a time when things would again feel normal and seamless. It came with its anxieties. I was confident that around the corner, there would be a morning when I didn't wake up in pain from a radiation burn, and my first thought wouldn't be about the fact that I was in treatment for cancer. Maybe, I'd be able to think about Samantha's graduation, Abbie's track meet, and Donald's baseball game. Maybe, when Brian picked up his camera, it would be to take a picture of me with long, messy hair. To get there, I knew that the only things that would help would be faith, patience, and time.

I had all three.

CHAPTER TWENTY-FOUR

The End or the Beginning?

Monday, April 23, 2012

MONDAY, APRIL 9, my last day, not only of radiation treatment but of treatments altogether, started off with a somewhat familiar routine. Mondays were normally the day I organized for the week ahead. But after I did the morning dishes and packed my bag for the gym, I methodically pulled various ingredients out of the cabinets and put them on the counter. The previous week, I'd been racking my brain thinking about how I could adequately convey my thanks to the staff at the Cancer Center on this last day. Nearing the week's end, I had *the* epiphany: "I know! I've got it! *Granola*!" Right? It seemed the perfect gift, because everyone I interacted with was very conscious of their health and as much as cookies and frosted desserts are decadent and appreciated, they defeat the whole healthy theme. I wanted my thank-you gesture to be different. Granola has all healthy ingredients, and it is so versatile! It could be put on cereal or yogurt or eaten plain, and I was going to make it myself with extra helpings of my secret ingredients: love and gratitude. Something homemade would express my feelings, make a statement, about how overwhelmingly grateful I was.

But as I stood in my kitchen looking at the oatmeal, soybeans, and flax seeds on the counter, I realized that somehow, homemade granola was about as lackluster as I'd feared. Granola? Really? Good Lord, what was I thinking? (Forehead slap!) It didn't say, "Thanks for the care – you are wonderful, and my interaction here couldn't have been more positive," as much as it said, "Hey, you have a black seed stuck in your teeth." Suddenly, I was underwhelmed at the prospect of walking in and disbursing a homemade cereal topping creatively packaged in decorative bags with ribbons. Had I come up with it when I was hungry? I put away the ingredients and sat at the counter, feeling defeated. I somehow knew this would happen. What seemed to be a great idea the previous week now felt grossly inadequate as I was heading in to see everyone for the last time. A thank-you card didn't feel like enough, but it was all I had.

I made a few cards for the front staff and the two radiation techs who treated me primarily. The cards had shoes stamped on them, and they said, "I'll miss shoe." It seemed appropriate, because the staff said more than once that although I would come in some days with a wig, other days with a scarf, and other days still with nothing on my head, the one consistent thing was my heels. They knew me for my shoes. It seemed fitting.

As I signed in for my last treatment, I was feeling strong. The receptionist who checked me in didn't realize it was my last day, but in casual conversation, I let her know it was. The three other check-in receptionists overheard and gave me the appropriate amount of "No way!" and "I can't believe it" comments to make me feel special yet again. They were good at that. I handed them the special card I made for them and could feel my composure slip. I told them I had to go or I'd cry, and I kept my smile as I headed out of the admission cubby. I couldn't make the goodbye TOO big of a deal, because I would have to pass by them again as I left. I didn't want it to feel like when you leave a party and say all your thank yous and goodbyes, give hugs and warm wishes and leave with the queen's wave . . . only to realize once you are outside that you left your keys inside on the counter, and you'll have to go through that awkward moment of encountering everyone again. (Um, or so I've been told.) Anyway, as I headed to change for the last time, I rounded the corner and heard one of them laugh. "Look! It has SHOES on it!"

I stepped into the changing room and did my normal change out of my shirt and bra, but before I slipped into my johnny, I looked at my reflection in the mirror as though to bookmark that day, as well as the intensity of my bright red breast and right clavicle. This daily tradition was about to end. Huh. I put my belongings in a locker and sat down and waited my turn. The more I thought about the finality of it, the more uncomfortable I got. I looked across from me in the waiting room, and two women, relatively the same age and stature, sat next to each other, both of them in matching johnnies with tied robes and blue pants. To cover up my melancholy mood, I asked them if they had called each other that morning to see what the other was wearing. A feeble attempt at mirth. Thankfully, they both found it amusing and looked at each other to discover the truth of the statement. Even more thankfully, I was called for the last time to the treatment room before it got any more awkward.

As the two techs escorted me to the machine, I gave them the cards I had made. I lay down, and we talked about how fast it had all gone.

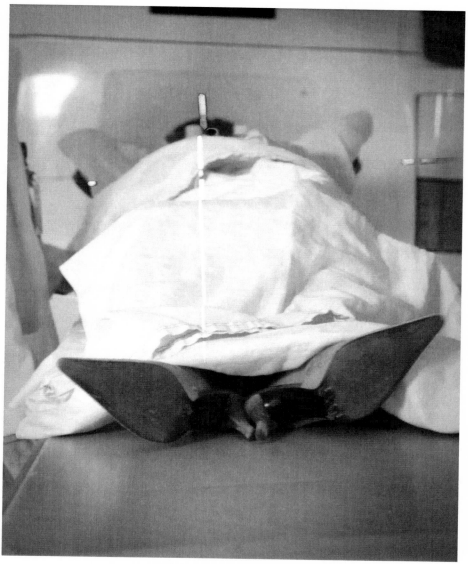

wicked witch of the west shoes

My last day, I got the "wet towel treatment," an added procedure that I got during every other visit. They put a wet towel over my breast to essentially "trick" the rays to irradiate the outermost part of my skin. One said, "What would your last day be without a wet towel?"

I had three different areas radiated at each treatment. One on my clavicle to irradiate the nodes that lay underneath and two angles on either side of my breast (extending under my arm) to cover the breast in its entirety. They adjusted me on the table and aligned my little tattoos with the laser beams. From there, they adjusted the table height and angle, as well as the machine that projected the beam, and called out the numbers and readings specific to me.

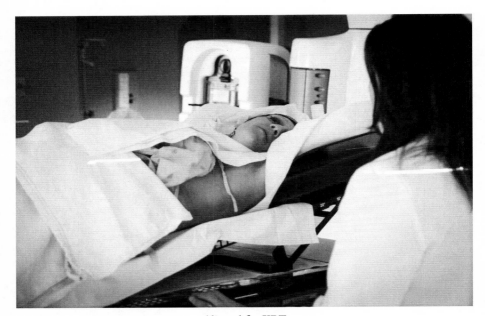

Aligned for XRT

They then left the room. Within fifteen seconds or so, I heard a constant, high-pitched beep. The beep lasted anywhere from twenty-five to forty-five seconds, and then it stopped with a CLUNK. The noise it made always made me think of that metal lever that controlled the electricity in "The Bride of Frankenstein." I was sure it was a simple electronic start/stop, but that was my mental picture. The women readjusted me like that three times, as they had the previous twenty-five other days, and before leaving the third time, announced, "Last time, ever." Then they walked out.

I was hyper-aware of my surroundings. I heard their footsteps leave. I waited a few seconds until the sound of the beep consumed the room. Beeeeeeeeeeeeeeeeee eeeeeeeeeeeeeeeep. CLUNK. Then silence. I lay frozen. I had heard it eighty-three times and it sounded the same each time, but this time, that sound meant the end of radiation. *Had it worked? Did this last dose kill off the last cancer cell that had tried to run off in my body like the last coward bad guy in a western who tried to run for the hills in the last second, only to be shot dead by the good guy?* I hoped so.

I was brought back to reality with the sound of cheery voices returning to the room.

It was the sound of the start of a new life.

The techs reported to me that I was to see the nurse for discharge instructions and then the doctor before I left. They gave me my "diploma" – a diploma-style sheet of paper signed by everyone who worked in the radiation department. It was all rolled up with a purple ribbon tied around it. They gave me a card also, and a gift from one of the local cancer support groups – "Amy's Treats" – for me to enjoy later. We said our goodbyes and promised to keep in touch.

I wanted to hear how long before C's daughter lost her first tooth. I wanted to hear how the cheerleading competition went for T's daughter. They genuinely asked about Don's science fair project, Abbie's track meet, and Sam's senior project. I wanted to hear about the updates on the wonderful little sound bites in their lives that had kept me feeling so healthy and normal, taking away the reality of why I was lying flat with my hands above my head as the rays worked their magic. Alas, this chapter too had come to an end.

I had been warned that I might feel anxious or depressed or sad at the end of treatment. I was mainly warned that it was a feeling of sort of dangling because the active part of treatment was now over. But nobody really warned me that although I would be making friends through treatment, as part of the end of cancer treatment, these friendships, by nature, would have to change. It reminded me of watching the highly volatile nature of both of my daughters' eighth-grade graduations. Everywhere you looked, there were girls crying and hugging and saying, "Don't ever change . . . keep in touch," as though they were moving to Mars and would never again see one another. The fear of the unknown was beginning to rear its ugly head for them. Life as they knew it – the security of the same four walls at the elementary school they had come to know and understand – would soon be a distant memory. They would have to venture out into the big world of high school, complete with responsibility and change. And they would have to start all over again at the bottom as freshmen.

I was feeling that unpredictable wave of the unknown as I walked into the waiting room for my discharge papers. I was leaving cancer treatment school to become a freshman of the "Healthy Adult University." One advantage of being a freshman is that starting over allows you to see things through fresh eyes and proceed forward based on what you learned in years past. I did have experience, after all, in the world of healthy living . . . it wasn't THAT long ago.

I walked into the waiting room and waited only a few seconds before I was escorted into the exam room, where my vitals were checked and I was to get my marching orders. The nurse came in, reviewed my paperwork with me, and reinforced my entire gamut of feelings. She handed me a stack of stapled papers with a basic summary of what I'd had done, accompanied by follow-up instructions for tending to my skin for the next week. She then asked me to sign on the dotted line. I took the pen and signed, wondering how many hundreds of times I had signed my name over the past eight months. I handed the paper back to her. *Huh. Done. Oh, wait . . . Done? Um, can I see that paper again? Did I read everything there? Am I numbed up so much that I just went through the motions here? Did I just miss something significant?* Up until now, with every signature, there had been another set of directions outlining the next phase of treatment. All I had now was, "We'll call you in a few months to schedule a follow-up with the doctor." *That's it?*

It reminded me of leaving the hospital with Samantha when she was born. The staff went over paperwork about follow-up appointments and restrictions and general baby care. I remember leaving the hospital with her in her car seat, walking out, saying goodbye, thinking, "When is someone going to stop me? I've never had a baby before! I don't have any experience with this. I am leaving looking all confident and ready, but I have NO idea what I'm doing, and I must have these people snowed, because they are all just smiling and letting me leave . . . somebody stop me!"

I may have donned my brave face as I signed these discharge papers at the cancer center, but I had no idea how to be a survivor. I had been all tangled up with structured movement within the web of treatment and now, someone had cut me loose, and I was dangling by a thread, about to fall into a realm where it would all be new again. The good news was that I hadn't been consumed within the web, and I had slowly and patiently wiggled myself free, but to what end? Closing this chapter of life was not what I had expected. I was now an official survivor. How did survivors begin this new life?

My radiation oncologist came in for one last check-in. He told me that my skin actually looked great for the end of treatment, but to be prepared for it to get worse for about a week before it started to heal.

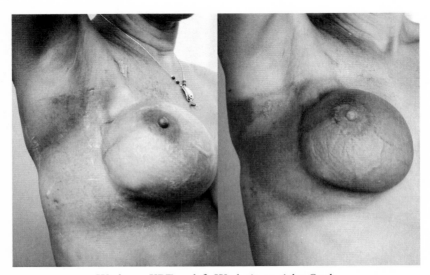

Week one XRT on left, Week six on right. Ouch

I should use lots of Aquaphor (a lotion to help soothe any burning), and if I needed more, to just come back in. He asked if I had any questions. That was a loaded question. *Sure. Thanks for asking. How much time do you have? Here's my question: Once I walk out this door and I'm done, then what? Can you answer me that?* Knowing my question was rhetorical, I just said, "I don't think so."

He stood up to end the visit. I gave him a hug and thanked him. He smiled and said, "You're awesome." I said, "You, too." That felt good. I wondered if he sensed that I needed something and threw that in. It didn't matter why at that point. I went back to the dressing room to change.

I vaguely remember leaving. I recall walking by the reception desk and then to the back, where I gave each of the receptionists a hug and a thank you. Healthcare is filled with hellos and goodbyes. But usually, I was on the other side as the healthcare provider. I didn't realize how it would feel here on the patient side. It was hard.

I hopped into the car, checked messages, and headed to the gym to keep up my regular routine. I was feeling overwhelmed and thought that a good run on the elliptical trainer would jolt my endorphins and get me over the hump. I was glad I did. But even still, as I drove home after the workout, a wave of emotion crashed over me. I cried on and off all the way home. But oddly, it wasn't because I was afraid or uncertain or sad. It was because I was . . . relieved. It was over. I did it. I went through a lot. I didn't die. I still had my humor. (Yay!) I was now on the "other side" of this. The tears felt great.

Once I got home, it was only a matter of minutes before Brian arrived as well. He walked in and said, "Congratulations! You did it! It's all over!" And I again felt overwhelmed with emotion. I cried on his shoulder, again with relief, but now also with acknowledgement from someone who had been through it with me. I tried talking about how I was feeling but had a tough time articulating. I felt as if I needed to debrief. When I worked on Med-Surg floors in the hospitals, if there was a code, or someone died or something big happened, all of the caregivers would make it a priority to get the chance to talk it through as a group at the end of the shift. Similarly, when I used to sing with a gospel choir, after a big concert, we'd all break down the equipment and head out to eat and talk about the show, the high points, and the energy. We would wind down within the company of those who had also experienced it. We all had the common denominator of "the event." Although we may have seen it or experienced it slightly differently, we'd all taken part, and it was great to be in the comfort of others who had been there, too.

The hard part now was that although my family and Brian had been there with me and were my comrades of a sort, it felt almost morbid to rehash it all. It was now in the past. How long would it be before I'd have normal stories to tell that didn't all revolve around treatment, aches, pains, and struggles? I knew those answers would come to me. Like the ups and downs of much of what I'd been through, when a new element presented itself, I needed a good twenty-four hours to absorb it and be in the moment before I could adequately deal with it. That was one of the more valuable lessons I learned about myself through all of this.

Brian took me out to dinner that night, and we spent a quiet evening together. Although I had wanted celebration with the end of chemo, I was content not to have anything over the top now. I was glad to be done, but I needed to sit with it before making any moves. A nice meal (that I didn't have to fix) in quiet company was just right.

Tuesday was a new start. First order of business? Back down to Boston to be "re-filled!" The "twins" were back! Well, OK they were back to being fraternal twins – they were about the same size, yet with they continued to disagree on which way was forward. Thankfully they were no longer "Irish twins," as they were when the left breast had 110 cc less saline than the right, with one clearly farther along than the other. I would no longer list to the right. My world was in better balance now, and I quickly came to grips with the fact that these girls would be with me for the next three to six months until it was time for final surgery. I left feeling confident. Symmetry is highly underrated, I always say. It was a good first step toward "recovery!"

As the end of treatment had neared, I thought a lot about doing something significant to draw things officially to a close. I wasn't ready to throw – nor did I want – a party, but I did know that I wanted something ceremonial to formalize it. So, Tuesday afternoon, I planned to plant a tree in the front of my house with my family. I have always loved weeping cherry trees, and somehow, planting one seemed to adequately symbolize this journey. There was, of course, the weeping – the branches all fall down as though they have been carrying the heaviest of loads and cannot possibly carry on. That was how I had felt at times through this treatment. But, in the spring, new life starts with beautiful white blossoms, followed by bright leaves that fill it in, exemplifying new life.

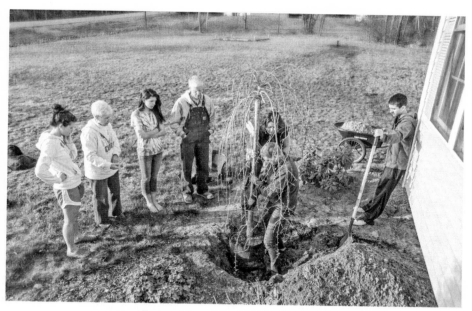

Digging the hole for the cherry trree

Mom, Dad, Anna, the kids, Brian, and I all donned various forms of "gardening clothes" (or work clothes, or work OUT clothes) and took turns digging, mixing the compost, and planting the new addition in front of the big windows of the great room. Mom and Dad had brought balloons over and put them on the railing and also brought over a dinner for us all to eat together. It was ceremonious, but not emotional – just succinct, meaningful, and representative of an end point, but also an equally new and healthy beginning.

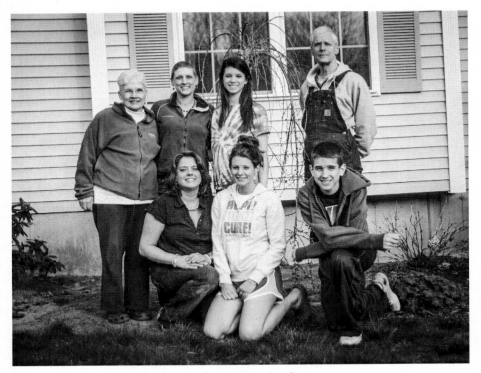

the family after planting the cherry tree

After dinner, Abbie presented me with a slide show that she had put together. She had organized a "Pink Out," where she had asked people to wear pink and take pictures of themselves and send them to her to show their support for me. More than eight hundred people responded! She told me that they had announced the "Pink Out" over the announcements at her high school for a few days before that Friday. She was so fearful that no one would be wearing pink. Instead, when she and Sam walked into the gym, there was a SEA of pink – pink hair, faces, accessories, shoes, and any other creative way to show support. (One young man had no pink clothes, so he put pink sticky notes all over himself.) Sam told her, "This is so much bigger than I imagined." The headmaster, teachers, and students had not let her down, and she felt a wealth of support . . . followed by the flood of pictures that arrived in her email, on her Facebook wall, and via text messaging on her phone.

Her slide show that night was more than ten minutes long and was put to music. The first song that played was Martina McBride's "I'm Gonna Love You Through It," and the last was "All Over Now." In the time it took her to upload all of the photos, more continued to flood in, but she wanted to present it to me that night. Those participating included students from five high schools in both Massachusetts and New Hampshire, members of gymnastics gyms (both from the one Abbie attended and from one of her gym's competitors!), staff from doctors' offices, students from middle schools, women I worked out with, couples we knew, family, friends, students from three colleges, coworkers from Old Navy, and more people from Florida, South Carolina, North Carolina, New Jersey, Massachusetts, New Hampshire, and Maine! I saw a few on Facebook and knew Abbie was up to something, but I didn't pry. She liked holding the cards and keeping me in suspense. She said she was going to add another song and the remaining pictures. I posted it on Facebook for everyone to view. It was a wonderful thing to experience the overwhelming support of so many people I both knew and didn't know, but I was also so proud of and touched by Abbie's efforts (with Sam's and Don's support, too) to coordinate something that went so big, so fast. And in a GOOD way.

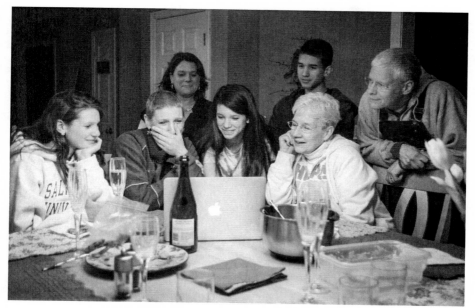

Watching the Video Abbie made for me

The days following the tree planting were calm and unremarkable. It felt eerily like the calm before the storm, you know, when things are just a little too still? Like that ten-second period of time when a toddler inhales silently, only to let out a blood-curdling scream. It left me wondering if someone was silently pulling back on a two-by-four, and it was about to smack me in the back of the head. But I presumed that was part of the uncertainty and the nature of healing after a life-changing event. I was told that although treatment was now behind me and I forged ahead, the next chapter of "life after treatment" would be just as challenging.

Cancer leaves marks. Emotional scars of fear and uncertainty. Physical scars from incisions, drains and radiation. But equally as deep are the metaphorical marks on my heart by those who touched my journey. Granola may have been a crazy idea; my healthcare team clearly deserved more than that. In retrospect, the only other gift I can think of that is worthy enough to mention would be to take the energy and attitude that they shared with me and pay it forward. I had been given a new opportunity to make a difference. But how do you package *that* in a plastic bag with a bow?

CHAPTER TWENTY-FIVE

The Descent

Friday, July 20, 2012

THE WEATHER IN New Hampshire had been typical, if there is such a thing. I classify it as "good gardening weather" – sunny for days in a row, followed by some decent rain. Thankfully, my days off corresponded with the nice days, and I was fortunate enough to start hiking again. I have fond memories of hiking as a child and young adult – backpacks filled with gorp, fresh fruit, peanut-butter sandwiches, and bottles of water. But sunny days and backpacks filled with great lunches don't necessarily make the hike a great one. Being physically prepared holds a lot of weight. I found that Brian's quote of "nothing prepares you for hiking except hiking" to be true as we set out on our first hike of the year. I also found it to be parallel with the time after cancer treatment. Nothing prepares you for cancer survivorship except surviving.

The past week, Samantha, Donald, Brian, and I headed to Tamworth, New Hampshire, to tackle the scenic, 3,500 foot, 7.6 mile, Champney Falls trail loop up Mt. Chocorua (sadly, Abbie was in Drivers Ed and couldn't make it). A scenic, moderate, six hour hike for those in good hiking condition. We all eagerly filled our backpacks with water-filled Camelbaks, bagels, peanut butter, and other various goodies and headed out to Tamworth for an awesome day hike.

Very early on during the hike, I determined that, without a doubt, I was "the weakest link" on this escapade and clearly would have been the one voted off the island. As the initial level trail dissipated and the ascent began, I followed the blazes as I frantically tried to keep pace with two kids (eighteen and twelve) and a-many-times-over, seasoned through-hiker. That was my downfall. I found it utterly depressing to think that the past three months of exercising four to five days a week at the gym had not better prepared me for this. I wondered what it would have been like if I hadn't exercised at ALL, and imagined I would be sucking wind so hard that I might inhale any nearby small defenseless wildlife creatures. I was breathing heavy. My legs were burning, and I was dripping with sweat, and Mother Nature decided to throw in a hot flash for good measure. I had to take off my sunglasses because they fogged up, and I could no longer see through them. But I found myself saying, "Six months ago I was sitting in a treatment chair with chemo running into my veins." This was far better than that.

As I questioned the physics and likelihood of spontaneous combustion, I realized that I was "bonking." I had eaten breakfast at around 8:30 am and had only replenished with water and an occasional bite of food. (Sidebar: Do not try to eat a dry, peanut-butter granola bar while climbing steadily uphill with a runny nose, gasping for air. It's a hiker's equivalent of the Bermuda Triangle trifecta.) My blood sugar was low, and my carb load of a whopping three-quarter cup of Whole Grain Cheerios consumed back at home had been depleted, most likely right about the time that I stepped out of the car at the base of the mountain.

At about 2:00 pm, we arrived at a flat peak and stopped for lunch. After eating, I felt one-hundred percent better. I was re-energized and scrambled to the top with a somewhat lighter load. (The weight of three fewer bagels, a container of peanut butter, and a half bag of Reeses Pieces is underrated.) The top was magnificent. It had been a cloud-covered day, yet the views seemed to go on forever.

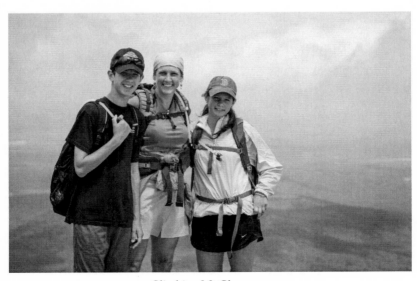

Climbing Mt Chocorua

As I stood at the summit, I remembered reading the activity restrictions sheet after my mastectomy. One of the items was no hiking until at least five months after surgery. *Pfffft. Hiking. Who the hell was thinking of hiking after a mastectomy, anyway?* At that time, I just wanted to know about when I could lift my hands over my head to shave my armpits . . . or get the dishes down to set the table. Or when could I go out and mow my lawn again. Hiking, golfing, Reverse Baby Cobra position in yoga . . . all of those things seemed like eons away. And yet here I was, nine months later, at the top of the mountain ready to conquer the world. I wondered which mountain I would hike next – what would be my next challenge? Of course I meant *besides* the impending descent down the mountain that was immediately facing me.

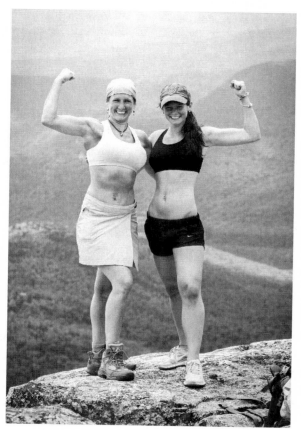

Sammy and I at the top of Mt Chocorua

The trouble with survivorship, personally speaking, is that when you have conquered something huge, and you know you have it in you and are feeling empowered, you look for the next challenge equal to or exceeding the last. Although I was *feeling* this, it wasn't until I visited my oncologist for a follow-up visit that she actually articulated it for me. Fortunately and unfortunately, after cancer treatment, there are not a lot of things that can rival "beating cancer." Cancer treatment was the ascent up the mountain. The gasping for air, the depletion of energy, the thinking that you are utterly exhausted and can't go any further . . . then you refuel, hydrate, and regain energy after a good rest and find that, lo and behold, you *are* able to make it to the top! That "worst part" is over. You did it! But wait. Um. Oh shit. It's not *really* over. Because, now you have to go back DOWN the mountain: survivorship. Although it is clearly easier than the ascent, the descent comes with its share of challenges, too. It's not as straightforward and seamless as it seems, even though it is clearly not as challenging as the ascent. If you go too fast or take on too much, you run the risk of falling on your face, twisting an ankle, or breaking a bone. The descent needs to be slow, careful, and methodical. As a survivor, if you try to resume your life as it was pre-cancer too quickly, you get tripped up.

I tried to ease myself slowly back into life. It has a way of feeding you things that keep your mind occupied, and I had a lot of good to focus on. Samantha graduated from high school. Abbie started Drivers Ed. Donald was selected to be the marshal for the graduating eighth-grade class. Yet somehow, I was restless. Somehow, I felt a change was imminent, that I needed "more," that something big was about to happen, and if I didn't make it happen . . . it might happen *to* me, the way it did with my original diagnosis. Although I never took my pre-cancer life for granted and was grateful for what I had, being a survivor does instill a seed in you that says, "Hey Lady, you have been given a second chance. So figure out what is good in your life and what you need to get rid of." *Gosh, what do I need to change? There must be something, right?* I was left feeling that whatever the change was, it must be monumental! I battled cancer and won! What would be next? Would I find a cure for the common cold? Would I uncover the secret to eradicate acne? Would I invent the perfect, calorie-free margarita? No, not likely. Finding the next monumental move felt like telling a long-distance hiker to take a walk around the block for exercise. *What? I just hiked from Georgia to Maine with majestic breathtaking views and now you want me to take a lap around the block for exercise? Where's the challenge in that? Why bother? That's crazy talk. NEXT idea, please.*

What is easy to overlook is that even though a walk around the block isn't as rigorous, it still contributes to taking care of yourself, just on a more realistic and normal scale. Expectations get skewed when you try to compare all challenges to "prevailing over cancer." But it's WEIRD pulling a colossal accomplishment out of the equation just to lower the bar. It's like having someone go in your wallet and find a fifty-dollar bill in the midst of a bunch of ones and say, "Oh, wait, that shouldn't be there; I'll take care of that." *But . . . wait . . . um . . . excuse me? That was mine . . . I earned it, and you can't just take it away.*

It is one thing to accept that you can reign over cancer. It's yet another thing to try to put that fact in its place and find the next challenge that yields a satisfaction level that comes anywhere close to that. It was difficult for me to maintain perspective.

Without that perspective, it was also difficult to embrace that I was restless during this phase. I felt as if I should be doing something significant and big, yet intuitively, I knew that really I should just enjoy what I had and put out the little fires that I longed for when I was going through treatment. How many times did I wish that the biggest hurdle I had was how I was going to fit grocery shopping in between work and picking up kids after their school events? Or that the biggest question on my mind was, "Am I going to be cooking dinner for three, five, or seven people, and who likes black olives and who doesn't?" Those concerns were a far cry from where I was emotionally during treatment, when I was dealing with fleeting thoughts about what I would say in the handwritten letters to my children that would be handed to them on their wedding or graduation days if the treatment didn't work, the cancer came back, and I wouldn't be around to be a part of those big events. Thankfully, I was back to the more mundane challenges and questions now. Identifying the olive lovers was back by popular demand. I tried to embrace it. Strangely, it was harder than it should have been.

Although the fear that the other shoe would fall if I didn't figure it out weighed on me, it also kept things in perspective and kept my eyes open – to new ideas, to the current beauty and good in my life, and to possibilities. These things kept me moving forward and kept that seed of fear buried and at bay.

Survivorship is a "learn as you go" process. I no longer woke up and thought of cancer, but it did still creep its way into my day at some point. I wondered about every decision I made and if it would be the "big one" that would clearly change my life forever. I thought about the next mountain I was going to climb and wondered if it would be bigger and better than the one before, or if it would be smaller and less majestic, but it would be a challenge nonetheless and contribute to my overall well being and help keep me strong.

Nothing prepares you for survivorship except surviving. You just have to keep doing it. Keep moving forward. Keep surviving.

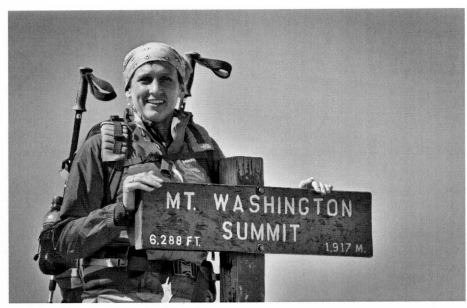

Later that summer I also climbed Mt Washington

CHAPTER TWENTY-SIX

Meeting the Twins

Saturday, November 17, 2012

THREE HUNDRED AND ninety days after my breasts were removed, I finally headed back to Boston to complete the final step of my cancer journey. I was going to have my "Expander Exchange," a surgical term that sounded as if I should be heading to an underground subway station in a trench coat to meet a shady, unshaven character for the sale of something illegal. In fact, it was where my expanders, the temporary, unnatural "goofy looking" saline-filled faux breasts that I had carted around for so long would be deflated, removed, and exchanged for permanent implants. "The final exchange." (It sounds like a title of a mystery novel, right?) Three hundred and ninety days later, I would finally meet the twins.

At one of my first breast cancer support groups, I listened to a woman my age cautiously share that she was going in for her final reconstruction the following week. Unfortunately, her announcement was followed up with the horror stories of two women who orated their dreadful experiences of their reconstructions. The leader of the group quickly jumped in when she heard the direction of the conversation and was able to refocus the discussion. As I watched the woman's excited expression deteriorate, I felt sorry for her. She looked aghast and slightly green around the gills. But the graphic surgical and post-op complications that shook her up didn't scare me as much as hearing her say that it had been more than a year since her original mastectomy, and she was only then going in for the final reconstruction. I sat frozen as my inner monologue took over: *WHAT? More than a year? Excuse me. Did she just say it's been more than a YEAR? Why on earth would she wait a year before having her final surgery? Pffttt! Thank God I won't have to wait that long. That is a ridiculous length of time to have to wait to be put back together.*

Just in case you are bad at math, three hundred and ninety days is almost thirteen months; it is just short of fifty-six weeks. And clearly more than a year. *Little did I know at the time, I too would have to wait more than a year for my final surgery date – despite my best efforts to be the model patient.*

I remember when the reality hit me that the final reconstruction date was not really in my control. When the oncology team told me at the beginning of this journey that the "process can take a long time," my glass remained half full. I thought, "Yeah, yeah. That may pertain to *other* people, but there is no reason why we can't move this along if I work *really* hard to stay healthy and keep on top of all of this healing." I mean seriously, I had heard TONS of stories about women who had their original mastectomies and woke up with their new implants and never even had to deal with expanders. Although I hadn't ever sat down and talked with a woman who had required expanders, I had never really heard a story about someone having to wait a year for reconstruction, either. Why would that even be? Because up until that point, I had heard what I had wanted to hear . . . that I'd be back to "normal" in no time. (Woo hoo! Watch me go!)

As you may recall, I had crafted a time line for my journey, as though *I* had control. All of the "healing time" in between treatments and phases was never part of my original equation and certainly did not gel well with my "Let's get this over with as soon as we can" outlook. I seriously thought that after radiation, I'd have to wait about six weeks (tops) for my skin to bounce back, and then I'd be ready to undergo my final surgery. Piece of cake, right? Not so much.

Going back to the six-week visit after I finished radiation, my plans first began to unravel as I stood in front of my plastic surgeon and proudly exposed my healing red right breast and its lumpy left cohort like a preschooler who presents a painting to the teacher and looks for praise. Her reaction and recommendation left me tearful and speechless. Although I was healing very well, it would be at LEAST three to six months before they would even consider the possibility of reconstruction. *What?* I had expected to hear, "Wow, you look fantastic! Let's have our scheduler get you on the books for your final reconstruction!" Instead, she took her fun-sucking straw and dunked it into my optimistic, half-full glass and took a big slurp. I sat, tearful, and confessed, "I feel very out of control right now." I tried to ask for further clarification, but I couldn't find my words; my mind had gone blank right after I heard "three to six months." *Good Gravy! That was two seasons away (I did the math in my head . . . May, June, July, August, September . . . OCTOBER?!) What about my plan to be bathing-suit ready for the summer? What about the ten-dollar-off-a-bra coupon I'd just gotten from Victoria's Secret that would be long expired by then? What about my desire to have pretty curves again and not feel as if people couldn't help but notice the awkward "elephants" on my chest?* Damn it. I was being handed the unwanted proverbial memo:

To: Tracy

From: Cowhorn Stage IIIb Invasive Lobular Carcinoma Treatment Guidelines

Re: Cancer Treatment Timeline.

Even at this stage in your recovery, due to circumstances beyond your control, cancer (and its corresponding treatment) will, yet again, be dashing your hopes. Your immediate concerns do not play a role in our current plan. Our goal is to give you the best possible outcome under the best possible circumstances. This does not, however, mean right now. We understand that you may not comprehend this right now, but we are confident that you will, in fact, thank us later. Thank you in advance for your trust and understanding.

What can you do but accept the news? Sure, for the first twenty-four hours, I ranted, cried, and stormed around, allowing myself to be mad, disappointed, and frustrated. But then, the realization came that it was just too much work to stay mad. And I needed to try to understand that these doctors knew what they were talking about. It might be my body, but I didn't have expander-exchange-after-radiation surgery personal experience. They did.

You may recall that when I went to Boston to have my left expander lessened before I started radiation, I inquired about other plastic surgeons. I wanted to be sure I had made the right choice. I visited with a second surgeon. He had rave reviews online and was known for his bedside manner. But I wasn't wowed the way I expected to be. He concentrated a lot on statistics, much of which outlined problems leading to "failure" of implants, perhaps to prepare me for all that could go wrong. After we talked, he looked at my expanders and his demeanor changed. "Oh!" he said, seeming somewhat surprised, "These look great." He felt confident that he could perform surgery so that I would be pleased with the outcome, but in fairness, he also mentioned that my surgeon had one very big advantage: she had done my original expander surgery and had a plan in mind at that time. He reinforced her abilities and his respect for her as a surgeon. I was very glad that I had gone to see him. The visit had given me the assurance I needed to feel comfortable with my original plan. To switch surgeons and introduce someone new at this stage of the game now seemed crazy.

Fast forward a year and twenty-five days. October 2, 2012. The final surgery day. I was not allowed to eat or drink anything after midnight. I was so excited that I was afraid I'd accidentally grab a drink or have a bite of something when I wasn't paying attention. Mom, Brian, and I headed out at 9:15 am to be in Boston by 11:15. I decided that I wanted to drive to try and keep my mind occupied and perhaps decrease my anxiety. (And we all know there's no better Zen place than in the driver's seat of your car as you sit helplessly at a dead standstill on Storrow Drive in Boston during morning rush-hour traffic.)

On the drive down, we had good conversations, but my mind was focused on the end of this phase of my journey. I felt tearful. Maybe, yet again, my trepidation was due to the anxiety of the unknown. Even though I had already been through what was said to be the harder of the two surgeries, this was the one I'd been waiting for for more than a year, and the outcome would be one I'd live with for the rest of my life. *What was I going to look like? Would I look anything like I did before my mastectomy? Anything would be better than the expanders, but would I look natural or would I wake up and feel embarrassed because she got my size all wrong? Would the recovery be as easy as I thought? What if my skin was too friable from the radiation and wouldn't heal or tore or had some other complication? Was I prepared to wake up and hear the recovery nurse tell me that there were complications and that they could do only one side and that I'd need a muscle/tram flap operation (a more complicated and invasive surgery using either my "back" muscle or muscles from my stomach) to fix what went wrong?* There was a lot to prepare myself for. I grappled with those fears and questions, but as I neared the hospital, I realized that I simply had to acknowledge them and leave them behind with the traffic on Route 93.

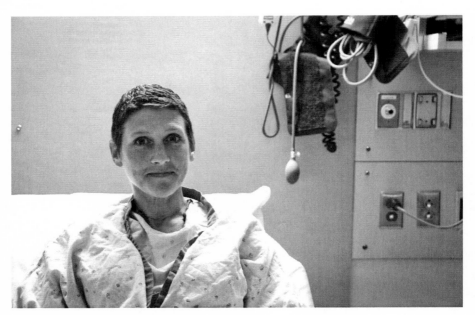

In the hospital for the last time, reconstruction, Finally!

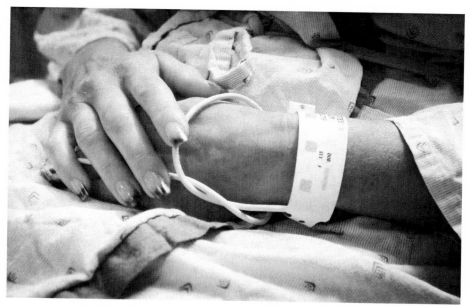

Ready and waiting

After "reporting in for duty," I waited for what felt like a long time. Even though I answered a plethora of questions for the nursing and pre-op staff, after I changed and Brian and Mom were able to come in and wait with me, it was hard to make small talk. We watched the clock. We watched the woman in the other bed wheel away to her surgery. We watched the "nature" pictures on the overhead TV repeat their loop every three to four minutes. I couldn't eat or drink anything to help kill the time, and Brian and Mom were getting hungry, too. At a few minutes before 1:00 pm, the transport lady came in to get me. Mom and Brian gave me a couple of "good luck" (not "good bye") kisses, and, as I was wheeled away, I heard Brian snapping pictures.

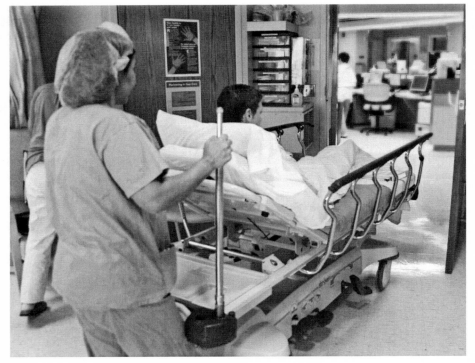

Wheeled away for surgery

Transport Lady and I went to the "express" elevators, where I was whisked with no stops down to the OR floor. It looked a lot like a basement. A familiar, yet uncomfortable, scent hung in the air. It was somewhat dehumanizing . . . the smell of sterilization and meticulous procedure. I wondered if this were the same place I came for my mastectomy, because none of it looked familiar. I was pushed through the ominous bowels of the hospital, where there were hallways of endless operating rooms. We passed OR after OR, and mine was the one at the very end. I was secured in a small waiting room outside of Operating Room 42.

Nurses came and checked on me. They let me know they were finishing up on a procedure in the next room where I'd be, and I would wait in the little bay until it was my turn. There, I'd see the anesthesiologist, have my IV placed (because of my chemo veins, I was NOT looking forward to that), and see my surgeon to get marked up, ask questions, get answers, and sign my consent.

I was happy to see the familiar face of my plastic surgeon emerge from the operating room. She was dressed in her scrubs and running sneakers. It was time to talk about the plan, sign the consent, and ask any remaining questions. We exchanged greetings. As she flipped through my chart, I told her that at midnight, I tossed and turned and thought of her, hoping that she was home getting a good night's sleep. She laughed and said she definitely had been. Although she looked happy enough, I asked how her day was going. I wonder how many people ask her that? I was hoping that on a one-to-ten scale, she was on the up side of seven or eight. She told me that she was having a good day, and it appeared genuine, so I was satisfied.

She asked me to stand so she could mark me up. I hopped off my gurney and stood exposed in front of her. With a fine-tip, purple marker, she wrote "yes" on my chest above both of my expanders, indicating that both sides would be operated on. She then drew a line with a tape measure at the bottom of my expander on the irradiated right side and extended that line across to under my left expander. Among a dozen other undesirable effects it leaves in its wake, radiation has a tendency to LIFT the affected breast. So, it was explained to me, that in addition to having the implant placed, my left breast would also be lifted and she would have to do some additional work to try to get my nipples to align. In addition, she said that she would remove fat from other areas of my body and inject it into the top part of each breast to create a more natural "slope." I asked where she was going to take the fat from, hoping that I'd get an early Christmas gift and it could be removed from that stubborn area on my belly that has graced my life since childbirth (aka the "pooch"). The area that taunts me and laughs at my efforts to tame it every time I do crunches or sit-ups.

She responded humorously. "Do you have any requests?"

I told her that I personally thought my abdomen would be a fantastic choice.

She smiled and nodded, but as I stood in front of her, she took a step back and tipped her head to the side as she looked at my waist. She put her hands on my hips and said, "Well, we could also go here and here," then moved down the back of my sides and continued, "Or here and here . . ." *Why did I suddenly have the urge to make a quick trip to the gym?* I didn't know if I should be grateful or offended, but what I *did* know was that I trusted her. I was no "fat-harvesting connoisseur," so I put my trust into her hands. She did this countless times a month. She was the expert, and I trusted her decision about where she'd point her liposuction wand to take my "donor fat."

As she wrapped up, I asked her if she could still videotape the surgery so that I could see what had been done. She said yes and that she would run back to her office to get her video camera. I know. Weird, right? I got a lot of funny expressions in response to my desire to see the video. Maybe it's a nurse thing. But to me, it would be strange to have no recollection of what went on for such a large chunk of my day while I was under anesthesia, especially after waking up with so much pain and such significant alteration to my body. I was curious and fascinated by how it would all happen. So, Netflix be damned, I have my own personal version of *Nip/Tuck* to watch (minus the sex, scandal, and illegal drugs). Bring on the popcorn!

The remaining staff ushered in one by one. There was the very kind anesthesiologist with his well-rehearsed routine that I could tell was one he could do in his sleep . . . all it was missing was the red flashing "Applause" light when he paused for my response. As he went through all of the things that I would experience (he described it as "a nice, long vacation"), another woman started my IV. Chemotherapy left her with few options, but after some initial, uncomfortable prep work, she slid a 20-gauge IV right in. She started the IV fluids and told me I'd be given meds to help me relax. Although I didn't feel anxious, at that point, who was I to argue? Relaxing was good. Bring on the drugs.

When everything was ready, they wheeled me in. One of the staff injected a shot of 100 percent pure delight and bliss into my IV. I don't remember much after that. I slightly recall being moved from the gurney to the OR table and seeing and feeling the oxygen mask over my mouth and nose, and hearing someone tell me to take deep breaths. I was breathing pure oxygen. Night night.

They started surgery a little after 2:15 pm, and I was told it lasted two hours. I awoke in recovery trying my hardest to battle the urge to sleep, but it appeared that someone had weighted my eyelids with lead. I knew that the sooner I got up and got going, started eating and drinking, and could pee on my own, the sooner I could go home. But I kept hitting the non-existent snooze button and fell back to sleep.

As soon as the recovery room nurse saw me open my eyes, she would say, "How are you feeling?" For all intents and purposes, that was a pretty straightforward question. But the transition out of anesthesia is a hazy and nebulous ride. Mind and body try to grasp reality while they're involuntarily pulled into a pharmaceutical Shangri-La. Hence, my answer to her question, *in my head* was, "Although I can't find my beer goggles, it feels like the jackalope is wearing mismatched legwarmers." (Seriously, it made sense at the time.) But thankfully, the answer that I uttered sounded more like, "I'm tired." I really didn't know how else to answer.

The anesthesia really does have to work its way out of your system. I knew the surgery was done, I was in the Recovery Room, it appeared that I had two breasts, and I was fairly certain that the Easter Bunny had stopped in. Past that, all bets were off.

Next questions: "Are you having any pain?" and "Are you nauseous?" Simple answer to both: "Only when I'm not sleeping." I tried a few times to pull myself up, roll on my side, or simply adjust my position. I knew there would be pain; it was normal and expected after any operation. But when I tried to turn, I expected the pain to be in my abdomen, the area from which I *thought* she was going to take the fat. No pain there. Huh. But very quickly, I figured out where the fat *had* been taken from. If you put your hands on your hips with your fingers forward and thumbs behind, it was RIGHT where your thumbs would be, on both sides. Then find the area on the outside of your hips where you would lie if you were on your side. Bingo. There were the other two spots. The good news was that I didn't notice the pain in my chest due to the bruising on my hips. The bad news was, no matter how I lay, I couldn't get comfortable.

The nurse tried to sell me her own little bill of goods – I was told that if I started to eat and drink, they could give me Percocet for the pain. Sigh. Look lady, this isn't my first rodeo. Even heavily sedated, I knew that sounded like a recipe for disaster, or at least for vomiting and constipation. Percocet on an empty stomach would make me vomit, yet keeping it down would bind me up for a week. And lest we not overlook the fact that all in all, it does very little to ease any discomfort. It appeared that dealing with the pain was still the least of all evils, so I said I'd wait on the pain meds. I did my best to be compliant and try to stay awake for as long as I could to drink the water that had been left at my bedside. I was thirsty for sure. She did give me some IV medication to help with the nausea, which coincidentally, put me right back to sleep. Sleeping was way nicer than vomiting.

We played the fall-asleep-wake-up game for a few hours until I was awake long enough to hold a reasonable conversation. At that time, I was offered graham crackers with my water. I was able to hold one down long enough to get the green light for transport to the post-op floor, the last stop before I could be discharged. Much to my dismay, the one thing that seemed to make me nauseous was movement. However, this unfortunate detail did not reveal itself until I was being wheeled on the gurney from the recovery room to the day surgery post-op unit. And even more unfortunate, the emesis bag that had been nestled in the crook of my arm in the recovery room had mysteriously disappeared from my bed and wasn't there when I needed it. How humbling to be sick and limited by both pain and nowhere to vomit. I do have to say that the up side was that it was only water, so it was pretty mild as far as vomit goes. The down side was that I threw up on my spare post-op bra and my other graham cracker. I hate it when that happens.

Once I arrived in the room, I got up to use the bathroom, cleaned up, and got the last of the vomiting out of my system. Mom and Brian came in and sat with me as I tried to sip on water and get comfortable enough to be able to face the ride home. It helped to be able to talk to them and have something to focus on; otherwise, I had no incentive not to fall back to sleep. It had been another long day for the two of them. Throughout the evening, they had been told repeatedly it would "just be a little longer." Thinking I'd be right along, neither of them wanted to go get a bite to eat, for fear they'd miss the call saying I was on my way. So, graham crackers aside, none of us had really eaten that evening.

After I used the bathroom, the gurney was taken away, and I was given a reclining chair.

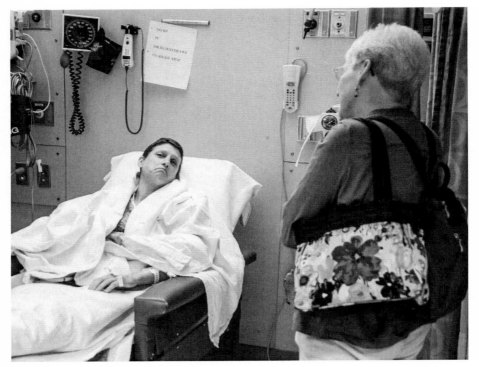

Post op chair

It was not comfortable, and I suspect that this discomfort is part of the "Master Plan" to get patients out. It worked. I kept thinking about the fact that I had an hour and a half ride home, and I just wanted to be in my own bed. I was handed a two-page set of discharge instructions. I read the first line over and again about twelve times. Reading plus post anesthesia does not equal comprehension. I was alert enough to scan through it to see if anything stood out that I didn't understand, but I wasn't together enough to ask questions. I would be on antibiotics for a week and was given a script of Percocet for pain. The nurse went over the instructions with me and asked me to sign the discharge paperwork. I had a little help changing into my clothes, and I hopped into a wheelchair for discharge. This time I had the emesis bag with me, which, thankfully, I didn't need.

The ride home flew by. I reclined the seat, and the hum of the car and the lasting effects of the drugs still in my system lulled me to sleep. It took only an hour and twenty minutes to arrive home safely.

Once home, I was battle weary. Up until that evening, I had tried to coordinate every big or significant treatment over the last year to coincide with the kids staying with their dad so that they wouldn't see me weak, tired, and vulnerable. Because Abbie had verbalized that she wanted to help, and Donald was OK with being home to help too, I decided to let them "help" for this last leg. (And although Sammy was away at school in Rhode Island, she stayed in touch all week and came home for the long weekend to be with me, too.)

I ascended the stairs into the kitchen from the basement slowly and methodically. I walked in to see a bouquet of flowers with pink roses, a red wine bottle with about one glass worth left in it. (I was instructed to avoid red wine, red grapes, and any anti-inflammatory drugs one week prior to surgery. Abbie knew which of those three I had missed!) A wine glass sat by the bottle, with a note in it that said, "Remember how one year ago you said that in a year you'd have your beautiful body back?"

In my darker moments after my mastectomy, when I had wrinkled piles of skin on my chest in lieu of breasts, I wrote that quote in dry-erase marker on my bathroom mirror. I looked at it each day. I knew that the odd expander look was only temporary. But I really, really needed the reminder. That day, one year and twenty-five days after my mastectomy, I could finally begin my healing with my new body.

I stood at my kitchen counter across from Don, Abbie, and Dad, with Brian behind me and Mom by my side. I saw the flowers and commented on the whole display and tried to remain positive and upbeat, but I clearly fooled no one. I was sore and too tired to make conversation. (Yes. You read that right. Too tired for conversation . . . I know! Red flag! When does THAT ever happen?) I just wanted to go to bed. How anticlimactic for the sweet-faced peanut gallery looking at me with relief, yet also worry. In the past, I'd had at least a day to get my bearings to be presentable to them, so I suspect they expected to see me happier now that it was all over. But, instead, there I was, with no sugar coating, standing wearily in front of them. At that point, I had to believe they were old enough to handle the reality of my post-op state, and I announced that regrettably, I really needed to get to bed.

Brian said that he watched their sober expressions as I headed upstairs with my mom. He felt as though he had somehow let them down. After all, he was the one they entrusted to look out for me, and yet he brought me back all stooped over, tired, and looking broken. They really didn't blame him. I think they were all – including Brian – a little shell shocked at the sight of me.

I have found that even as an adult, when I'm sick, or vulnerable, I still just want my Mom. She helped me get changed and settled in after I brushed my teeth. It was difficult to find a comfortable position. I wasn't allowed to sleep on my stomach (nor could I, due to pain), and the bruising from the "liposuction" still ruled out any comfortable position on either side or on my back. But it was mostly the moving that hurt. Once I was positioned and could lie still, it was OK. I slept through until about 4 pm, when I knew I needed something for pain. Regular Tylenol helped.

I was told that this recovery would be much easier than it was after my mastectomy. The physical part was – the overall pain was significantly less. But the restrictions were almost identical to the first time around, which may well have been exceedingly worse than before. Simply speaking, I felt better, so I wanted to do more, sooner. But: No driving until my post-op appointment, wear the utility bra around the clock except when showering, no lifting more than ten pounds, no lifting my hands above my head, no activity that would cause my new breasts any angst, no vacuuming, no lawn mowing . . . for *four to six* weeks. At least. Gah!

So, even though I was awake and up and about early Wednesday morning, Brian had to drive Donald to the bus stop. I waited until they were gone for a moment alone. I was anxious to finally see the twins. Similar to the timing of my mastectomy, the reveal wasn't until the following day, when my head was clearer and I could comprehend what I was seeing. I went into the bathroom and stood in front of my big mirror for the "unveiling." This was the moment I had waited one year and twenty-six days for. I unzipped my utility bra and pulled it off my shoulders. In front of me was a bruised and swollen set of unfamiliar breasts – a version of the new me. Their shape and positions were vastly different than the expanders – they now had soft curves and slopes and no jagged edges. As expected, the left breast had a bandage covering the same incision line as the original surgery, yet also up and around the top half of the nipple. There was also a bandage underneath both breasts. I didn't know why it was under the left, but figured it had something to do with the "lifting" part. There were two small Steri-strips above each breast that covered the quarter-inch incisions where the fat had been inserted. There was quite a bit of bruising. My nipples were not perfectly facing forward as they once were in their natural state, but they were at least fairly even. (Let's just say that they no longer screamed "Marty Feldman eyes.") I knew a lot of swelling needed to go down before I could get a more accurate picture of what they were going to truly look like, but from what I could see, they were keepers.

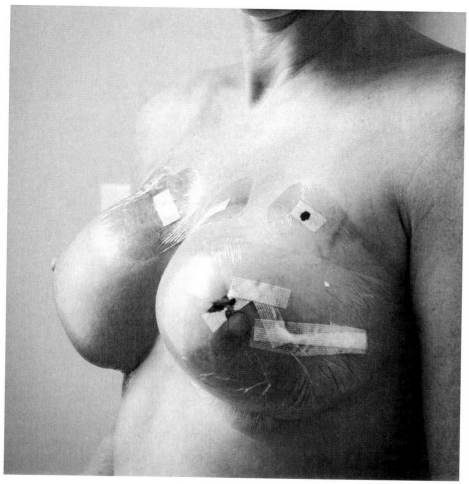

Two days after surgery

Strangely, as I stood there, I found it difficult to remember the intricacies of what my breasts looked like before. *Was that weird? How could I have something be a part of me for forty-two years and not remember them now?* It felt like getting a new haircut and expecting to see yourself with long hair when you look in the mirror, and you're shocked to see short hair, but as soon as you see it, you forget that you ever even HAD long hair.

What I do remember is that in my mid-thirties, I considered myself fortunate to have found the perfect bra. I wore it (in varying colors, of course) night and day, knowing that gravity was the enemy, and I didn't want the girls to go down without a fight. This perfect bra was generous, fastidious, and steadfast. (Not to mention pretty, and, given the right color, could be downright sexy, too.) It pulled every ounce of each boob into its snug, full cup without any embarrassing overflow spilling out over the edges. I was packed in tight. (Yet surprisingly, with an adequate amount of room for the essential tube of lipstick or other various and sundry last-minute items that might need stowing.)

So, as I stood braless, looking at this new body reflecting back at me, I noted a few things. For starters, I could see the ribs below my breasts – novel. They had been sheltered for years and were now exposed due to my recent surgical adjustment. These new breasts were higher (or perhaps "perkier" is the right word) than before, and, lo and behold, they looked similar to what my old ones had looked like in my "perfect bra." But their shape was different. It's hard to explain. They were one-hundred percent better than the expanders . . . so for that, I was thankful. But although they were nice, they really didn't feel like mine yet. Maybe it was sort of like driving a new car off the lot. As exciting and new as it is, the car doesn't really feel like yours, because it is unfamiliar. Its full capabilities are unknown and yet to be discovered. I saw the girls in their glory standing before me, but I had yet to figure out their full potential. *Would they hug the curves? Would they be good in the rain and snow? Could they go zero to sixty-five in ten seconds?* I would soon find out. It was time to fasten my seatbelt and take them for a ride.

One of my best friends had gone through treatment for breast cancer a year before me. At the end of her treatment, I bought her a sexy, black bra. To me, it symbolized a rite of passage. A month post-op, at my final follow-up appointment, the medical assistant took down the last of the bandages. I got clearance to go back to my regular activities, and I *finally* got the green light to wear "regular" bras! At long last, it was my turn! It had been more than a year since I'd been able to wear or buy a bra that was not the sports variety – the kind that pulled over my head or looked like "Helga's Utilitarian Tit Sling" with ties, snaps, zippers, and Velcro. Finally, I could don a simple, pretty bra that hooked *in the back.* So, on the way home from Boston, Mom and I hit Victoria's Secret so I could be officially measured and try on different styles . . . and use that ten-dollar off coupon I'd been hanging onto. I discovered that after the swelling subsided, my new size was actually one cup size smaller than it was pre-cancer. I suppose the payoff was that although I was one size smaller, I would be eternally perky. It was all good. We walked out of Victoria's Secret with a few new bras, representative of a returning normalcy that made me feel as if things had officially come full circle. Walking out the door with that pink bag in hand, I felt as if it were really over. It truly felt like my rite of passage.

So now, it appeared that the last "official" phase of treatment was complete. Mastectomy, chemotherapy, radiation, healing, and reconstruction. I was now entering a new phase that I hadn't before thought of as an actual phase; "living as a cancer survivor." The phase that would continue until it unassumingly phased itself out.

I heard that if all goes well, each day gets easier. This would be a chapter where, I hoped, I would think less each day about what I've been through and more about all that might lie ahead – but in a good way. I found that, for a while, a cancer reminder would creep its way into my head at some point every day. But it also got easier each day to let go of the fears and scary or bad memories. Each morning when I took a shower, my new breasts looked less foreign and more like my own. My scars were fading. The physical pain of the reconstruction gradually abated, and I could now lie on my stomach once again. (Something I hadn't been able to do since before my mastectomy.) I could get dressed for work and reinvent uses for the plethora of scarves and pashminas as accessories for my neck and shoulders instead of a head covering. I could go to the gym and work out and feel normal in an exercise tank. Now, when people asked me how I was, I could report that I was well – cancer free for more than a year. Even though I didn't know this for sure, nothing catastrophic happened to lead me to any other conclusion. I was optimistic and had faith.

Will I make it past the five-year mark where the chance of recurrence decreases significantly? I don't know. Only time will tell. But up until that point, all I can do is live each day appreciating all that I have. I can reflect back on all I've been through and the blessings contained in each experience – support of the community, family and friends that came out of the woodwork, quality time I was given with people who visited me as I healed, received treatments, or was driven to and from appointments. I will dream of the future – spending my days with friends and family, watching my children grow up and graduate from high school and college, then get married and have their own families. I will look forward to being a part of every day I am given with health, energy, and a grateful heart.

Truly, what did not kill me made me stronger, more grateful, and richly blessed.

EPILOGUE

Taming My Bellows

YOU KNOW, IN general and overall, life after cancer is pretty darn good. I mean really. What could be better than having a slew of treatments, tests, procedures, and medical expenses comfortably behind you? Everything has been completed with flying colors, and I have officially been given a clean bill of health. Oh yeah – and hair, and better still, energy! It's a new beginning!

So, you might wonder, what do I do first? Well, funny you should ask.

My answer was once, "Get back to life as it was before." It was all I thought about. *Just get all of this behind me so I can get back to normal.* But the truth is, my life will never be the same. The normal I knew is long gone. I may have the same physical surroundings, house, car, clothes, job, friends, and family, but what I know about life has changed. I lived in a world where I never thought cancer would or could happen to me. But it did. As a result, my sense of security changed. Although I have gained a renewed appreciation for what I have and what is important to me, I am now intimately familiar with a new level of fear that I quietly carry with me wherever I go. Because of that, my official answer to the question above is, "Find a balance between life before and after treatment." Once that is established, carry that balance, that peace, as gracefully and yet as enthusiastically as you can. And move forward.

In order to live happily, I had to find and accept that balance. Trying to figure out what to worry about, what to give attention to, what to let go of, and when to act are all part of that. And a lot of it has to do with looking deep within, trusting your instincts, and knowing that you need to make the most of today. As cliché as it sounds, you really DON'T know what tomorrow will bring. Looking *within* for acceptance, happiness, and peace is important. But it is not always easy.

I had two eye-opening experiences with trying to seek outside validation as I tried to accept my post-cancer body. One materialized when I went to see my general surgeon for my one-year, follow-up appointment. As a reminder, at the beginning of my treatment, he was the one who provided the much-needed insight to help me decide whether to have one or both breasts removed. That was one of the biggest decisions I'd ever have to make . . . and he was one-hundred percent there to help me. Because it was such an important decision for ME, I lost sight of the fact that the feeling wasn't ever supposed to be mutual. Why would it be? I was not his friend or relative. I wasn't a patient with whom he had developed a special bond because of extensive treatment or surgery. Yes, he knew me by name, and I was a familiar face, but to put it bluntly, I was simply just another female patient he followed up with a year after a breast-cancer diagnosis.

Up until that appointment, I had not exposed my new breasts to anyone but a close inquisitive and select few. Other than Brian, my general surgeon would be the only other male who would see the end result of my reconstruction. Up until this appointment, that was a personal and conscious decision. But when I walked into the exam room, I no longer saw this man as a surgeon responsibly following up on one of his patients. He had somehow morphed into the first *man* to see my reconstruction other than Brian. *Holy Crap!*

Although it sounds insecure to say, I think I was subconsciously looking for some sort of validation about how I looked through the eyes of a man, someone who was not my partner. Yes, Brian did tell me how beautiful I was and how my new breasts looked great. He had watched their painstaking transformation through every stage. However, not to diminish its importance, I wondered if his positive accolades stemmed from his general supportive nature or the obligation of a good boyfriend. Like a mother who praises a young daughter for the "great job" she did at tee ball when, in fact, she ran to third base first after she hit off the tee with her helmet on backwards, made designs in the dirt when she was supposed to be watching for the ball, and was only really playing to get a slushy at Cumberland Farms after the game. Sometimes, being supportive means you accept that things are what they are. Whatever Brian's motivation was, I was grateful. But I was now faced with hearing an unbiased opinion.

At my appointment, unaware of my expectation, my surgeon stood the course and remained nothing but professional and um, well, did I mention professional? After the physical exam, he told me that everything looked good and recommended that I lift my right arm when I massaged lotion into the scar tissue to help decrease the pain and to help release the right breast, which was still "tight" from surgery. He then handed me my paperwork, said that he didn't need to see me for a year, and asked if I had any final questions. *Wait, what? YES, I had questions! What were his thoughts? Did I miss the part where he said, "Your surgeon did a great job," or "Everything turned out very nicely," or even a simple, "Nice symmetry"? Even my female oncologist said what a nice job my surgeon had done.* I wasn't looking for anything inappropriate, just some acknowledgement that, professionally speaking from a testosterone-driven human's point of view, I should be happy with the surgical work done. Coming from a male surgeon, it would have meant a lot. But, alas, no.

I realized on my drive home that it was an unfair expectation for me to think that he would have provided that validation for me. It wasn't his role or responsibility. I had to start just believing that everything looked good to ME and that was all that mattered.

To be honest, I continued to struggle with that. Don't get me wrong. It's nice to hear people say, "*You* look great," because I know that it is the politically correct thing to say. Occasionally, my mom, a close friend, or female co-worker would say more specifically, "Your boobs look great," which always makes me smile. It also makes me think, *a good boob day can be as meaningful as a good hair day, but ninety-nine out of one hundred times, it goes completely unrecognized.*

Anyway, my second eye opener happened one day after a gospel concert I attended. On my way out the door, I ran into the band's bass player. (I knew him because I used to be a part of the choir he played with.) He's a man of few words, with a killer sexy smile. I hadn't seen him in a while, and he mentioned he'd heard that I'd had cancer. He asked how I was doing and what I'd had done. After I told him the Condensed Readers Digest version, he subtly glanced downward, and very tactfully and honestly said, "They did a great job." It was meant – and received – as a compliment, and it was as unexpected as it was refreshing and validating. I thanked him for saying so. It took a lot of courage to be so honest. My mom, who overheard, said, "That was sweet of you to say. I'm sure it means more to hear that from someone other than her mom." (*Did she just say "sweet of you"? I guess I've reached a new point in my life where a man compliments my breasts in front of my mom, and it isn't awkward. In fairness, it* was *sweet.*)

I realized on my way home that afternoon that as sweet as that comment was, as a whole, similar comments are VERY few and far between. If I was going to wait for such comments for validation, well, who knows how long I would have to wait? It drove home the reality that it was really time for *me* to accept how I looked. I knew all along that others' opinions didn't matter. What others think of me is none of my business, right? It should matter to no one but me. It reminded me that my bust was, figuratively speaking, only one very small, physical part of me . . . and certainly not nearly the most important part. It was a strange turning point for me, but I am glad I had it.

Validating moments aside, making it to the other side of cancer treatment is a triumphant victory. On the big scoreboard of life, I am seeing (in bright lights): TRACY: 1, Cancer: 0. I am proud, confident, and utterly grateful to claim this conquest. But I often can't help but wonder if the devil isn't feeling defeated by my conquest and subsequently looking for revenge. I wonder if the last cancer cell floating around in my body has been overpowered and wrestled to the ground, or is it riding around on its little cancer cell broom cackling, "I'll get you my pretty . . ." as it searches for the hidden source of estrogen it needs to grow big enough to make its reappearance. In that case, it might look more like Jack Nicholson peeking through the broken door in *The Shining*. "Heeeere's Recurrance!". In EITHER case, I sometimes get a looming feeling that just when life is good, maybe it is *too* good. Or, as Frieda says, "Someone is pulling back on the two-by-four," and it's just seconds from hitting me on the back of my head.

I have been told that this sense of fear or paranoia that something scary is about to be uncovered is normal. I suppose knowing that brings a low level of comfort – it means I'm not alone or just being a drama queen. The fire of fear that was once an inferno has essentially burned out, leaving behind a subtle glow of embers. Every so often an unexpected wind blows a little oxygen onto that fear, and its coals emit a bright orange glow. And yes, there are events that cause that fire to ignite as though it had been primed with a bellows or fed with straight gasoline.

A few catalysts have increased my worry level and reignited my fire – the anniversary of my diagnosis, appointments, any new alteration in how I feel, and watching a friend's journey with cancer come to an end.

Realizing that the anniversary date of my diagnosis was affecting me came to me as an epiphany. In July 2012, I started getting antsy and anxious and I didn't understand why. Brian was getting ready to make his annual pilgrimage out to Burning Man. He leaves for around two months every summer to head west to Black Rock City, Nevada. It was right after he left in 2011 that I had my initial biopsy and was diagnosed. So the next year, as the time neared where he was packing up to go, the days were also at their longest, the flower boxes were overflowing with petunias, and the windows stayed open all day and night, filtering in all of the wonderful sounds of summer. I had been hyper-aware of these surroundings when I was diagnosed. Brian's departure that summer compounded feelings that I hadn't defined. My increasing anxiety was spurred simply by the sounds and sights of this time of year – it was like walking into a house that you haven't visited in years, and just the sight of it makes you suddenly reminiscent of past events. Or you smell something that triggers a memory. Sometimes the memory is good; other times, not so much. It wasn't really the cancer itself that scared me. It was the anxiety of all of that unknown ahead of me. So, the actual anniversary date wasn't as significant as the summer season itself was (I simply thought, "Wow, it was a year ago today"), because the compilation of my surroundings brought me back to how anxious and uncertain I felt when it all started. It sort of felt like experiencing a death on someone's birthday. A normally happy occasion suddenly has a negative connotation attached to it.

I think that on some level, a follow-up appointment will shake even the bravest of people. Going back to the surgeon who told you about your diagnosis or to the oncologist who knows the intricacies of cancer is nerve racking. Like I said, I never thought cancer would happen to me in the first place. And although I had cancer, I was also lucky. I am alive and well! But demons creep in and make me wonder, *how often can I be lucky? When I go in for this follow-up appointment, will my labs reveal some subtle detail that isn't obvious on the outside? Is feeling well a false sense of security?*

At my follow-up appointments with my oncologist, I'm usually asked a list of questions and then have a physical exam. I don't have breast tissue to be evaluated, so I no longer undergo mammograms (sayonara, boob pancake machine!). There is no reason to perform further full-body scans unless I have other symptoms. *But what symptom is worthy of concern? A swollen gland? Forgetfulness? A lump? A cough?* So, how do they know that everything is ok for sure? With no actual "tests," the logical result is that if you are feeling OK, you have to assume that all is well.

So, devoid of further testing, you have to just "take that to the bank" and rest well, knowing the doctors have no glaring concerns. I've tried hard to focus on the good, because to focus on anything *but* the good makes me a little crazy . . . OK, more crazy than I am already.

This leads me to my third catalyst: discovering any alteration in how I normally feel. I will preface this by saying that as a nurse, I do start off ruling out the totally illogical possible diagnoses. However, after filtering through the logical answers as to what is most likely ailing me, every *other* possibility then enters my head, and before I know it, my imagination has me admitted to the ICU on a ventilator. *Headache? I never get headaches . . . how bad **is** this one? Get me a mirror . . . are my pupils equal and reactive? Could this be an aneurysm that has sprung a leak and is slowly bleeding into my head, only to be stopped by an emergency Med-Evac flight to Boston for an aneurism clipping? Or, wait . . . am I just dehydrated from working out in the sun all afternoon and not drinking enough water?* It's what I do. I like to refer to it as being hyper-aware of all of my bodily functions. Some refer to is as being melodramatic. To-may-to, Tom-ah-to.

In the end, with almost every symptom, I usually wait it out to see if rest or an over-the-counter painkiller helps. The problem with this methodology is that I waited for the lump on my breast to get at least acorn-sized before I had it checked out. I "waited" to see if it would go away. It didn't. Now, I don't really know how long is *too long* to wait. There are no definitive symptoms for breast cancer recurrence. So, does this mean that I have to wait until my skin and the sclera of my eyes are turning yellow before I'll know that there is something affecting my liver? And by then, is it too late? Every twinge can make me think,

"What was that?" Every cough that doesn't abate can be metastasis to the lung instead of allergies, and every ache in my leg can be from bone cancer instead of the result of the new exercise program I am doing. It takes a conscious effort to back the truck up and keep things in perspective. I am doing it. But, I was burned once . . . and it is sometimes difficult.

This leads me to a recent event. It was my one-year, post-treatment appointment with my oncologist. Things were fine. All systems go. I was switched over from Tamoxifen to an aromatase inhibitor (AI), Anastrozole. This medication has slightly better studies outlining a decreased chance of recurrence, but can only be given to post-menopausal women. The side effects that are most troublesome are the joint and bone aches. I was instructed to let my oncologist know if they became too much to bear. After one year post-treatment, I graduated from Tamoxifen, which felt like a milestone.

The good news with this new medication was that I was no longer having multiple hot flashes every day! I hadn't realized that it was the medication that had been driving the flashes to this extent, I just thought it was part of the rapid menopause transition. The dwindling of the flashes happened simultaneously as the new side effects of the AI kicked in. The side effect *du jour* was now bone aches. The up side was that it made me forget, or maybe not care, about the hot flashes. After about a month, the aches had abated and only seemed to be noticeable first thing in the morning.

However, just when things seemed to be going along famously, I noticed some "mild spotting." (Cue the ICU and ventilator images.) *Good Lord! What does this mean? Was it from the new medication? Was I transitioning out of menopause? Were my ovaries confused? Had the cancer spread?* First word of advice: DON'T try to Google what it means! The truth of the matter is, although spotting isn't "normal," it could be from a plethora of different things, many of which are benign. All I could focus on was that it was new and wasn't normal. As if my worried mind didn't already have me planning my funeral. Before you could say, "hysterosalpingo-oophorectomy," Google had me "drinking the Kool-Aid" and exploring ovarian cancer signs and symptoms and planning out my next chemo schedule. I decided to call my oncologist to allay my fears.

Fortunately, I already had my annual gyn exam scheduled for the following week, so I asked if I should just wait for that or if I should get in sooner. She was comfortable with me waiting. But, she said, "Just to be safe," she would call my gyn doctor and have her do a pelvic ultrasound the day of my appointment. It was probably nothing. She asked if I would be OK with waiting the week, and I said yes. I thought I would be.

As it turns out, up until the day of the appointment, I was unsettled. Although the spotting stopped after four days, I was worried that it was a symptom of something going on that I couldn't see on the outside. I had lab work done the morning of my appointment (to check my hormone levels) and then the ultrasound. The last time I had an ultrasound was when I first saw my breast cancer. I found myself trying to research online what a normal ovarian/uterine ultrasound would look like, but it was an impossible mission. It was WAY beyond my abilities. I would have to trust that I'd know soon enough.

As I lay on the table, I watched the screen where the scan was displayed. The two ovaries looked very different to me – one was dark and small, and the other was light and misshapen. The ultra-sonographer took multiple pictures of my uterus. She clicked, measured, and marked off different views, and I asked how she knew what to look for. She gave me a vague response: "Because it is what I do, and I see it every day." *Was it me, or did that sound like the answer, "Because I'm the Mom"?* It was a fair answer, but I guess what I had really wanted to hear was, "Ms. Matteson, I don't say this to just anyone, but this looks like the healthiest ovary/uterus combination I've seen in weeks!" (If I had a nickel for every time I heard *that*.) She wasn't going to spill what she knew or what she saw, so I had to resign myself to the fact that I'd have to wait until my appointment later that day to get the results. It was only a couple of hours away, but those hours felt like an eternity. I am not ashamed to say that I popped a Xanax after I left to minimize my brain spins.

Finally, at the follow-up appointment a few long hours later, the first thing my gyn doctor did was review the ultrasound results with me. Calmly, but a little perplexed, she said that a normal uterine lining should be a half a centimeter. Mine was measuring *one and a half* centimeters. This was sometimes the result of the Tamoxifen. And, I had read, can sometimes (but rarely) lead to cancer. *More cancer from the cancer treatment. How cruel is that?* She suggested that we do a biopsy of my uterine lining to know for sure. She had everything on hand to do it right then and there. Without hesitation, I said yes. I couldn't live with the anxiety of not knowing for sure if there was something more happening. The biopsy would give us definitive answers. Within five minutes, a pinch and a poke later, it was over. The results would be back by Friday. It was Tuesday.

I tried to let the worry go. I tried to give it up to God and put it in His hands. But I kept taking it back and worrying. I tried to prepare myself for the worst, but still, I wondered why I was still a mess inside. I thought about my summer, my work, my family, everyone who would be affected by more treatment. I knew if it WAS cancer, I could do it. I'd done it once already. I even tried to reassure myself by saying that if it was cancer, it was most likely a separate primary site and not metastasis. That was good . . . but that would have to be staged too . . . and what if it was a late-stage cancer this time? And why, WHY couldn't I put this in perspective? I was a wreck. After three long days of waiting, all pathology was reported as normal. It was most likely from the Tamoxifen. The news was both a relief and exhausting.

Well, the fourth and final fire catalyst played a big role in why. On June 1, 2012, a friend with whom I went through simultaneous treatment passed away from metastatic breast cancer.

In February 2012, near the end of my chemo, my friend Jen from the Navy said she had a friend, Lisa, who was also going through treatment for breast cancer. She asked me if she could share my journal with her. Jen had been following my entries and felt that perhaps Lisa could appreciate some of the humor in this virtually humorless ride, as well as have someone to talk to about the blessings and frustrations of cancer. I said sure. I also looked her up, and we connected on Facebook.

We kept up with one another and sent email messages back and forth starting that February. We compared notes about our hair (or lack thereof), medications, various treatments, and how we were doing emotionally. She "got it." She understood how scary it was to entertain the thought of metastasis. She could relate to the craziness of the medications. Although we had never met in person, we were in the same unfortunate club. She too was a prayerful woman. Her "I'm right there with you" emails comforted me.

Eight months later in October, I saw on her Facebook wall that there were a lot of prayers being sent her way. I sent her an email asking what was going on. Within minutes, she responded and said that she had just found out that the cancer had metastasized to her lungs and lymph system. She told me that she had been given two months to a year to live. I had been about to head to work when I saw the email. I spontaneously burst into tears and cried all the way to my office. This cancer stuff had just gotten real.

Oddly, I realized that I couldn't put my finger on exactly *why* I was crying. My sadness went beyond words. I was *so* sad for her. But this news also triggered so many emotions for me. We cancer patients all face our own mortality. We run full speed toward the edge of that cliff, only to stop in the nick of time to peer over the edge at what lies beneath. It's an unthinkable fall. And the premise of that fall is where everything in life shifts – priorities, planning, living for what is truly important. Hearing her tell me that she was now in Stage IV breast cancer felt as if we'd been holding hands together for a while running toward the edge of that scary cliff, and then, at the last second, I stopped and let go of her hand. *Oh, my God! Lisa, wait!* I didn't mean to, nor did I want to, let go. Although she thought she'd stop too, because of circumstances beyond her control, she couldn't. Yet she looked back at me and smiled. Our journeys were now going in different directions. She was truly happy that I had been able to stop. She was happy that I was doing well. Survivor's guilt. It's not, "Why me?" It's, "Why not me?"

I realized that I no longer knew how to comfort her, because although I had peered over the edge of the cliff, peering over and falling are two very different things. I THINK I know what I would do, but I don't know for sure. And trying to picture myself in her situation in order to relate to and support her was unfathomable. It made me lightheaded and a little nauseous.

Everyone's journey is different. For every one person who encounters a recurrence, there are so many more survivors. In fact, there are survivors everywhere! The natural advice given to someone like me who is worried about recurrence is:

focus on the positive. Honestly, it is great advice. Yet somehow, I can't just dismiss someone with whom I have this unique bond, someone with whom I have come to love and respect. Together, we have been in a shipwreck. The life raft has come, and there's only one seat left. I was at the right raft at the right time. And although I've been pulled onboard and am thankful to have the seat, I can't seem to find comfort in all the others on the life raft with me. That is because all I see are the people floating in the water who can't be helped and are less fortunate due to circumstances I will never know or understand. It leaves a deep scar. I *can't help* but feel sad for the ones who can't be saved. And not understanding why I am so lucky is hard. And scary.

So, as much as I want to concentrate on all of the success stories, I experienced a loss. A woman, only six years older than me, with kids younger than mine, has lost her battle. This is my bellows. A simple gyn exam becomes exacerbated, because I am still trying to sort through the "whys" of this unfortunate occurrence. It becomes a delicate balance between why and why NOT me?

The thing is, you just never know. Random things happen to people that they never see coming.

When I was fifteen or so, I worked for a little Greek sub shop called "Pete's Roast Beef." One evening just after closing time, Pete, Nick (Pete's brother), and I heard a car pull into the parking lot. The engine cut and two doors slammed closed. Moments later, we heard the sound of stones crunching beneath the feet of someone approaching the building. I was washing the dishes and looked over to see Pete's eyes as wide as golf balls.

He said, "What do you want?"

I turned and saw a handgun make its way through the door, attached to a man with a ski mask, followed by a man with a knife in his hand and a nylon stocking over his head.

One of the men held the gun to my head and instructed me to get down on the floor. I was easily persuaded. They proceeded to rob us. *This is it. I'm a goner. I am only fifteen years old and about to be offed for the price of a lousy day's worth of subs.* Although it would've totally been worth taking a bullet for a slice of Pete's baklava, I doubted that it was worth it for the money we had made that day.

We were instructed to stay on the floor and count to one hundred before we got up. I counted out loud, "seventeen, eighteen, nineteen . . ." while Pete and his brother talked about what to do next. But, apparently as an afterthought, the rookie robbers realized they forgot to disconnect the landline. They came back and ripped the phone off the wall. This was back in the day where no one but James Bond had a cell phone. We were left wondering if they'd make a third visit. "Twenty-five, twenty-six, twenty-seven . . ." They didn't.

But before I could reach "one hundred," I had been introduced to a new level of fear.

There are two points to this story: (1) You are sometimes a victim of circumstance and are simply at the wrong place at the wrong time, or something unforeseen happens over which you have no control, and (2) When that happens, you have to continue to put one foot in front of the other and move on. You can't let fear paralyze you and stop you from living life. Yes, the sound of stones crunching made me a tad jumpy for a while after the holdup. But it happened for a reason, and I grew from the experience. Instinctively, I reevaluated what I could hold onto and what I could let go of. The love of an authentic Greek salad? Yep, that's a keeper. Making a dollar-fifty an hour at a sub shop and risking my life? Nope. That one had to go.

Almost thirty years later, my cancer journey has also allowed me to grow, and instinctively, now that the worst is behind me, I have reevaluated what is important. The scars that started out as swollen, red, and painful have faded, and the memories of how hard it was to go through treatment are still there, but not as tender to the touch. Those scars have become a subtle reminder of my strength and of all of the good that has come of it.

I look at the women in my life whom I secretly admire who have had breast cancer and live full lives now: Dianne, Shannon, Charity, Bridgette, my grandmother, Carol, Sister Sue, Debbie, Jean, Marty, and Susan. We are all so different and handled things in our own ways. Some experienced FAR worse than I, and others breezed through it with little to no fanfare. Mine is a story that has only one voice. Not everyone feels or experiences everything I did, but maybe they can understand the uncertainty or anxiety I felt.

My own valuable lessons are these:

1. Cancer is "udderly" a Cowhorn experience. Going with the flow made things easier, especially because the rules might, could, and did change on a moment's notice.
2. Some days, as Sister Sue told me early on, it's not just one day at a time, but it can be "one breath, blink, and heartbeat at a time." Although every day meant I was one day closer to finishing treatment, some days were clearly harder than others, both emotionally and physically.
3. I learned how to ask for and accept help from those who wanted to do something – it helped not only me, but them, too. I will remember how helpful this lesson was for me to learn, so I can reach out to others in need.
4. For me, thank the good Lord, humor, irony, and sarcasm still prevailed through this journey. I allowed myself to laugh. From eyelashes that came unglued around noon and dangled impatiently in my line of sight for the remaining half of my workday, to receiving coupons for twenty-percent off of bras that claimed to make me two sizes bigger (how scary was that thought?), to the ideas of assembling a "bra-jazzeling" kit to bring a little sunshine to the ugly, surgical post-op bras, humor lived on, and I was very grateful.
5. Prayer continues to be a powerful thing. Appreciating and watching for the gifts of each day can be hard when you are challenged. But God gave me

these gifts in the form of exceptional medical staff and friends who brought meals, drove my kids to games, played guitar with me, sent cards, prayed for me, checked in on a regular basis, and made me feel "normal," supported, and loved. And for all of that, both then and now, I count my blessings daily.

6. All beautiful things come from a place of suffering.

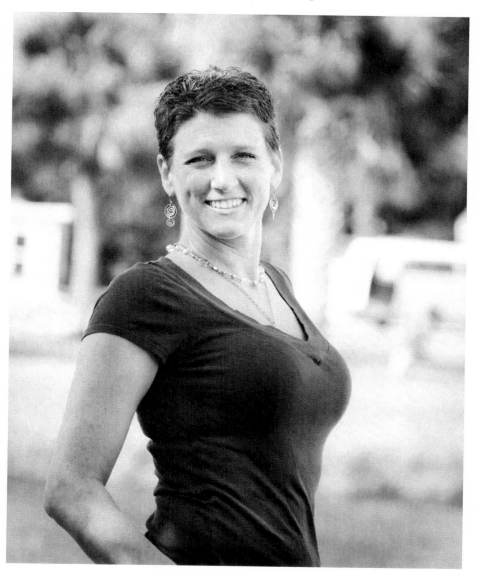

After all is said and done

Edwards Brothers Malloy
Thorofare, NJ USA
October 30, 2013